Career Development for Nurses

Opportunities and Options

Career Development for Nurses

Opportunities and Options

Jane Sanderson
MA RGN
Clinical Nurse Adviser, Leeds General Infirmary

Scutari Press
London

A division of Scutari Projects, the publishing company of the Royal College of Nursing.

First published 1993

British Library Cataloguing in Publication Data

Sanderson, Jane
  Career Development for Nurses
  I. Title
  610.73

ISBN 1-871364-92-2

Typeset by Action Typesetting Limited, Gloucester
Printed by Athenæum Press, Newcastle-upon-Tyne

Contents

Preface

This is a book about ideas and action, contacts and useful information: a career guidance service that can be used anywhere in the world. It is not intended to be an in-depth discussion of individual occupations or employers, but a taster.

Nursing is an exciting, rewarding and very diverse occupation, and nurses have many skills that can be transferred usefully into new situations and new careers. I hope to have reflected this in the content of this volume and wish every reader success in their chosen careers.

Introduction

The collapse of the conventional career (Davies 1990) quietly but effectively marks the profession's recognition that nursing career patterns have changed. Employment trends in nursing suggest that career breaks, time out, part-time employment and mobility within nursing are increasing. Employment trends within nursing have been changing rapidly for some time.

Handy (1985) indicates that within employment generally, as greater productivity is expected from each individual, fewer people will be needed to do the jobs. As more people become available to work in different capacities (part-time, job share, self-employed) the number of jobs is decreasing. In the health care industries and professions individuals are being expected to take on more diverse activities, and greater caseloads, to accept more responsibilities, to be more highly skilled and flexible.

Some nurses are choosing careers outside the conventional structure or moving into careers that are allied to nursing. Some return at a later date. The Royal College of Nursing survey (Waite & Hutt 1987) indicates that sixteen per cent of nurses had a second job and that one in five of the nurses surveyed had changed their jobs within the first seven months of 1986. This same survey notes that over half the nurses surveyed had left the National Health Service, were considering leaving or had given up work altogether. The 1992 survey (Seccombe & Ball 1992) notes that one in four nurses surveyed had changed their job in the previous twelve months. The same survey indicates that one in three of the sample had career breaks at some stage in their working life prior to the survey.

The message in this is clear for both nurses and nursing. Nurses need to plan their careers effectively in order to make the most of opportunities within their working lives. Nursing needs to provide career development guidance to individuals if it wishes to retain or attract back an enthused workforce.

The enormous range of opportunities available to nurses is often underestimated. Sources of information about these opportunities are very scattered and sometimes inaccessible. This volume attempts to provide access to a wide range of opportunities and give direct contact with the many employers and institutions. Such a vast subject is difficult to cover completely; therefore, this volume is not exhaustive but aims to give reasonable coverage of relevant topics. Salaries and other details that are likely to change considerably have not been included. Addresses and other particulars are subject to change, so readers are advised to make their own specific enquiries about the particular opportunity that attracts them.

The title Registered Nurse, for all nurses on the UKCC register, now replaces 'enrolled' and 'registered' in their previous usage. Within the new registered nurse status there are two levels that replace the former two-tier system. First level nurse refers to the former registered nurse and second level nurse to the enrolled nurse.

The differences between the opportunities for first and second level nurses remain the same and the titles registered and enrolled are still the most commonly used terms.

REFERENCES

Davies C (1990) *The Collapse of the Conventional Career.* London: English National Board.
Handy C (1985) *The Future of Work.* Oxford: Blackwell.
Seccombe I & Ball J (1992) *Motivation, Morale and Mobility: A profile of qualified nurses in the 1990s.* Brighton: Institute of Manpower Studies.
Waite R & Hutt R (1987) *Attitudes, Jobs and Mobility of Qualified Nurses.* A report for the Royal College of Nursing. Brighton: Institute of Manpower Studies.

Section One

The Future after Qualification

1

Immediate Choices and Expectations

On paper, the number of available opportunities must seem bewildering to the newly qualified nurse. Apart from the very large number of organizations by whom the qualified nurse could be employed there are numerous specialties. Many of these specialties may not have been covered during nurse education.

In reality the situation is somewhat different, the choice being confined to the jobs that are vacant at the time of course completion and the personal constraints upon the nurse at the time: for example, transport to and from the place of work.

Many nurses, therefore, find themselves in jobs that may not necessarily be their first choice, but will help them gain some initial experience.

THE IMMEDIATE CHOICE

At the point of qualification, and even before, identifying a job vacancy that might be suitable becomes the priority. Factors influencing the choice of job include personal circumstances, career pathway preferences, preferred specialty, the people with whom you are going to work and support issues. With this in mind it is worth analysing your position before you make the next move. A careful analysis of the situation is worth undertaking each time you change your job. This issue is covered later in Section One.

The jobs that are closest to your ultimate aim are the most obvious ones to apply for, but even those jobs which are not immediately linked to your ultimate goal may suit you for other reasons. Care of the critically ill patient may not be the immediate choice of a nurse who wants to work with children or the elderly person, but the job itself could enable the nurse to gain other skills which may help at a later date.

Weigh up the benefits and disadvantages of each job vacancy in terms of your ultimate aims and the skills that you will need to gain.

EXPECTATIONS

Both the employer and employee will have a set of expectations from the new contract of employment.

The newly qualified nurse as employee should expect a period of support during which he/she begins to learn about the role of a qualified nurse and the duties involved in the new situation. In addition to this a knowledge of the specialty will be required. PREP outlines a period of four months' support from a preceptor for the newly qualified nurse. Currently most good employers offer some kind of support period during which the new nurse is assigned to a more experienced nurse. These programmes range from an informal arrangement to a full course, depending upon the organization and particular managers. Before you accept a job establish the nature of this support. Do not confuse support for newly qualified nurses with the normal induction programme. Normal induction programmes are usually available to all new starters in the workplace and have a strong emphasis upon orientation and specific details relating to the working environment.

The employer will have certain expectations of the newly qualified nurse, one of which will be participation in the support process and acquisition of the skills and knowledge necessary to ensure safe and competent practice as quickly as possible.

Experienced practitioners moving from one post to another should aim to seek employment where there is a strong commitment to professional development. The nurse moving from one discipline to another may benefit from targeting organizations that offer specialty development programmes to help the new starter. These development programmes are not to be confused with the induction programmes, and can often be negotiated on an individual basis.

2

Post Registration Education and Practice

The Post Registration Education and Practice project (PREP 1990) is seen as the profession's response to the individual's professional development. Designed to commence at the point of qualification, PREP envisages a continuum of development over a nurse's career span. In time, with increased specialist skills, further education and practice the project suggests that the nurse will work towards becoming an advanced practitioner. The sequence of events is as follows.

Primary Practice

Primary practice is the period following registration. During the period of primary practice the initial four months are undertaken with the guidance of a preceptor; the preceptor helps the novice to apply knowledge to practice and work towards agreed learning objectives. By the end of the initial period of support the novice nurse should be competent to take responsibility for his/her practice in cooperation with others. During the rest of primary practice the qualified nurse continues to gain experience and confidence within the workplace. Undertaking a six-month programme of education leading to a recordable qualification, such as the National Board specialist courses, can lead to specialist practice status.

Specialist practice (enhanced practice for midwives)

Nurses and midwives practising at this level have a recordable qualification of not less than six months' full-time study and provide leadership to others. Teaching, support and advanced clinical care are seen as part of the roles at this level, and skills, knowledge and practice are developed further during this period. Community health care nursing courses are at this level and include the following six areas of practice:

- nursing care of adults;
- nursing care of children;
- nursing care of the mentally ill;
- nursing care of the mentally handicapped;
- nursing care of employees in the workplace;
- nursing contribution to the promotion of community health, child protection and health maintenance.

Advanced practice

Advanced practice status can only be obtained by practitioners who have undertaken a six-month specialist course, achieved further experience at specialist level and then completed an advanced three-month recordable qualification. Advanced practitioners lead nursing, ensuring high standards of care and undertaking initiatives such as research and practice development.

Throughout the stages of professional development nurses undertaking further recognized study will accumulate credits towards diploma, degree and advanced degree status. This will be administrated under the Credit Accumulation and Transfer Scheme (CATS) (see Section Three for a full description).

RE-REGISTRATION

During the working life of a qualified nurse the nurse is required to undertake five study days every three years. This can be undertaken as full- or part-time study and must fall into the following categories.

- Practice development (e.g. study of practice elsewhere).
- Care enhancement (e.g. quality assurance studies).
- Reducing risk (e.g. health education).
- Patient, client and colleague support (e.g. counselling courses).
- Education development (e.g. ENB998/997).

Certificated evidence of study in one or some of the above categories is required as evidence in the re-registration process and as part of the nurse's professional portfolio.

RETURN TO PRACTICE

Nurses returning to work within the profession who have completed less than 750 hours or 100 working days in the previous five years must undertake a return to practice course such as the ENB 902. Return to practice is discussed in more depth within Section Two of this volume.

UKCC PERSONAL FILE

The UKCC personal file, used for recording and reflecting upon personal data and experiences, also contains a professional profile. The contents of the professional profile will be used for the purpose of verification when the practitioner re-registers every three years.

KEEPING A PERSONAL PROFESSIONAL PROFILE

The UKCC document on the post-registration proposals contains a proposal which states that 'all practitioners must record their professional development in a personal professional profile'. The profile itself is to contain details of formal education, an assessment of developmental and educational needs and an action plan to meet these needs. Part of the philosophy underlying the rationale for a professional profile is the belief that professional people reflect upon and learn from their practice, experience, education, training and other achievements.

The professional profile as a record of practice, experience, education, training and other achievements is more than just a curriculum vitae or career résumé. It helps the individual to evaluate retrospectively, reflect and plan for the future. This process of formally recording progress should help each nurse to plan their career and development with more structure and to present their case to potential employers more effectively.

Profiling includes the documentation of skills gained and contributed to particular jobs held by the individual. Details of special projects and advances made in a professional capacity, in particular those which are practice-based, are also contained within the profile. A record of private experiences that contribute to professional life, such as voluntary work, are an important part of any profile. Education and training are also recorded within the profile.

A vital part of any profile is the record of self-assessment and an action plan for the future. The goals and action plan for the future are based partly upon self-knowledge of personal and professional strengths and weaknesses combined with a vision for future development.

Part of the profiling process may be undertaken with a mentor, manager or preceptor who is able to help the individual assess themselves, their needs and direction.

Ultimately the detailed content of the profile is likely to be decided upon by yourself, your mentor, manager or preceptor as based on its professional relevance at the time of discussion and recording. The UKCC has indicated that it expects individuals to take responsibility for this particular aspect of their development.

With the above in mind nurses should begin to accumulate evidence of further study, projects and practice development ready for insertion into their profile. A folder containing letters of attendance, notes of projects and other developments could be a useful start for each nurse.

USEFUL READING

Brown R A (1992) *Portfolio Development and Profiling for Nurses.* Lancaster: Quay Publishing.

Green M (1991) *Post Registration Education and Practice Project.* London: UKCC.

Rogers J & Maggs C (1992) Distinguishing characteristics. *Nursing Times,* **88**(19): 54–6.

UKCC (1992) *Register.* London: UKCC.

3

PREP and Career Development Pathways

PREP is aimed at existing as well as future practitioners and is for all grades of qualified nurses. PREP has obvious implications for career choices and should help to develop individuals remaining within the profession. Opportunities within education, management and clinical areas now have more clearly defined pathways. PREP does, however, recognize that not all individuals who train to be a nurse will remain within the profession: a significantly high number of people leave the profession each year. A few of these individuals choose alternative career directions; some leave to have families or for other personal reasons and return at a later date. Return to practice is addressed by PREP. Individuals returning to practice after a break of five years or more, and who have been employed for less than 750 hours or 100 working days within that time, will need to undertake a return to practice course such as the English National Board 902. Return to practice is addressed in Section Two.

PREP addresses the future of nursing and health trends. It envisages a scenario in which nursing consists of a single first level qualification from which the qualified nurse develops into a competent practitioner with increasing expertise. Qualified nurses can begin to mould their qualifications and experience (past, present and future) to fit into this pattern. The process of consciously considering development within the PREP framework should help nurses to develop their career into the future more effectively.

Career pathways begin to develop after the initial period of support and during primary practice. It is therefore advisable to attain qualifications which are recognized by the UKCC and can be transferred under the credit accumulation and transfer scheme.

Other professional, further and higher education bodies are addressing the need to have credit accumulation and transfer schemes. In future it is possible that individuals who take courses allied to nursing may be able to transfer elements into the nursing scheme. At the time of going to press, all of these schemes (some of which are described in Section Two) are in the early stages; it is therefore difficult to be specific about particular organizations and practice.

PROFESSIONAL DEVELOPMENT WITHIN CLINICAL PRACTICE

For the newly qualified nurse the primary aims should be to gain as many skills as possible in order to be able to practise safely; much of this is likely to be done under the guidance of a more senior nurse who is clinically competent. The novice nurse should be more than a consumer of expertise. He/she may be able to contribute new ideas, recent research and a fresh approach to some aspects of care using their recent training to full advantage.

Development as a primary practitioner beyond immediate novice status can come in a number of ways. Some nurses may wish to consolidate their experience in the same clinical areas and move on more rapidly into advanced skills. Others may choose to work in different areas for a while in order to gain broad experience before specializing.

The overall service requires both nurses who are specialists and nurses who are able to turn their hands to a number of things within care delivery teams, therefore both of these routes are equally useful. Ironically, immediate promotion within the clinical setting is usually dependent upon the depth of specialist clinical expertise, but in the long term nurses applying for many senior nurse posts may find that employers want broad experience with some evidence of specialization.

The more advanced primary practitioner may find that his/her development includes the guidance of others and involves being a preceptor and primary nurse. At this stage in the clinical development other options such as management and education begin to interface with the role. The primary practitioner who is a senior staff nurse will find that the role includes a responsibility for education and deputizing for charge nurses or sisters in their absence. Most nurses begin to formulate preferences at this stage and, accordingly, to develop some relevant skills while in the clinical setting.

Development within the clinical setting can be continued through the role of sister/charge nurse and into that of the clinical nurse specialist. As an expert practitioner, the nurse can expect to become much more specialized as a clinical nurse specialist or may opt to take on a role such as adviser, which would still involve clinical input but may be much more general in emphasis. These roles are discussed in more depth in later chapters. Beyond specialist practitioner the qualified nurse can continue into advanced practice.

Further education, which includes clinical specialist courses, study days and conferences, are all essential for the nurse's development process. Attendance on study days and conferences are not only important for maintaining a professional profile but part of the advancement process within PREP.

PROFESSIONAL DEVELOPMENT WITHIN EDUCATION AND TRAINING

As a primary practitioner the qualified nurse is likely to be able to gain credit for undertaking further courses, such as the ENB 998/997 Teaching and Assessing, which is then used as a basis for developing programmes that are relevant to the clinical area. This initial stage of development within education and teaching is likely to be an experimental one during which the nurse discovers and perfects various methods and styles of teaching and educating others. This early process will help to develop skills and determine future direction for the individual concerned. Many qualified nurses may choose to confine these skills to the current workplace and develop in different ways. A few will choose to move out of immediate clinical practice into an educational role.

A variety of roles can be used as part of the development process. A number of organizations have roles which combine clinical practice with education. These roles include clinical tutors, who seem to be predominantly placed in colleges of nursing, and nurses with roles such as clinical specialist/tutor who are often ward- or unit-based. Both these roles are likely to have different amounts of clinical input to educational input and will vary from individual to individual. These types of roles may allow an individual the opportunity to move with more ease from the clinical setting into education.

Other roles within education and teaching are those of in-service training officers, professional development leaders and nurse tutors or lecturers.

All of these roles require further education and training as part of the development process. PREP requires nurse teachers to be graduates with an advanced qualification and a relevant teaching qualification. Further details of these roles and access to information can be found in Section Two.

PROFESSIONAL DEVELOPMENT WITHIN MANAGEMENT

The first contact with management skills is likely to be during practice as a primary practitioner. This is developed further in the roles of charge nurse/sister.

For nurses who wish to remain within direct line management in a clinical area, the most obvious route is into nurse management. The qualified nurse who chooses this path will need to be able to divorce himself/herself from the day to day clinical details and to concentrate energy on more strategic work such as planning, recruitment development issues and ensuring smooth administration. Development beyond the immediate clinical setting into management requires further education, which involves management courses. Beyond nurse manager the qualified nurse can advance into management at higher levels within organizations and theoretically to the very top of the profession.

Some nurses may choose to develop themselves in a different direction, moving into management of a variety of non-nursing situations but still within the health services. It is not clear how PREP relates to this type of development, since all PREP's emphasis is upon the development of the nurse who remains within nursing.

USEFUL READING

Baker J (1988) *What Next – Post Basic Opportunities for Nurses.* London: Macmillan Education Ltd.

Benner P (1984) *From Novice to Expert: Excellence and Power in Clinical Nursing Practice.* California: Addison Wesley.

Cormack D (ed) (1990) *Developing Your Career in Nursing.* London: Chapman and Hall.

Green M (1991) *Post Registration Education and Practice Project.* London: UKCC.

Johnston M A (1992) A personal task. *Nursing Times,* **88**(14): 29–31.

4

Employment

Prior to the start of a new job after the offer and acceptance of a post, both the employer and employee enter into a contract. The contract of employment can be verbal or written; in either case it is binding but it is usual for the formal contract to be written. Employees can expect a written contract within thirteen weeks of beginning employment. The contract should state the main terms and conditions of employment, including the length of notice required to terminate a contract.

Termination of contract can be by a number of means:

- termination by the employee;
- termination by agreement between the employee and employer;
- termination of the contract by the employer.

Termination of the contract by the employer can be by means of:

- dismissal; or
- redundancy.

The employer and employee have three sets of obligations to each other in the work situation.

- Contractual obligations and requirements.
- Legal obligations and requirements.
- Moral obligations.

Contractual obligations and requirements

Just as employees are not supposed to breach their contract by absenteeism without good reason, the employer is bound by contract to pay the agreed salary and cannot pay the employee less without agreement or notification. Both parties are expected to honour the contractual agreement in all respects.

Legal obligations and requirements

In addition to the contract employers have a set of obligations to employees in general which, for example, may include the provision of protective clothing (under the Health and Safety Act 1974). Other examples include the legal obligation not to discriminate between employees on grounds of race and gender or to dismiss an employee unfairly.

Employees have the obligation, for example, not to act in a negligent fashion (as discussed in Legal Aspects of Nursing, page 17). Under the Health and Safety Act employees have a duty to wear the clothing provided, when necessary, to help them ensure a safe working practice.

Moral obligations

Moral obligations are not formal requirements but are, nevertheless, still obligations. Not so easy to define and not usually written, these moral obligations include loyalty to the organization for whom you work and support and respect from the employers to employees.

FURTHER INFORMATION

Specific reading on the law of employment can be obtained from *Law of Employment* (Selwyn 1988) and *Rights at Work* (McMullen 1984). Advice covering the issues of employment can be obtained from the health care unions and personnel managers.

As part of regulating behaviour within the organization, many organizations have grievance and disciplinary procedures. These can be obtained from the personnel department.

INSURANCE

In addition to the statutory National Insurance Contribution many organizations have pension funds. Employees of the National Health Service can contribute to the superannuation fund, or opt out of this scheme in favour of a private pension plan. Individuals looking for a pension fund can find details of independent brokers and insurance companies in the local *Yellow Pages*. You are advised to choose an adviser/company that is registered with the regulatory bodies, Financial Intermediaries, Managers and Brokers (FIMBRA) or Life Assurance and Unit Trust Regulatory Organization (Lautro). Details of registered companies and advisers can be obtained directly from either FIMBRA or Lautro.

Other major issues that are likely to concern the employee include maternity leave and pay, along with sick leave and pay. There are a number of excellent leaflets on these issues which can be obtained from the local Department of Health and Social Security. Your employer/personnel manager may have some copies, and your general practitioner's surgery may carry a supply for information.

REFERENCES

Department of Health and Social Security (1974) *Health and Safety Act*. London: HMSO.

McMullen J (1984) *Rights at Work – a Guide to Employment Law*. London: Pluto Press.

Selwyn N (1988) *Law of Employment*, 5th edn. London: Butterworths.

USEFUL READING

Evans R & Durward L (1984) *Maternity Rights Handbook*. Harmondsworth: Penguin Books Ltd.

Upex R (1980) *Law at Work – Dismissal*. London: Sweet and Maxwell.

USEFUL ADDRESSES

FIMBRA,
   Hertsmere House, Hertsmere Road, London E14 4AB.
Department of Social Security,
   Richmond House, 79 Whitehall, London SW1A 2NS.
Lautro,
   Centre Point, 103 New Oxford Street, London WC14 1QH.
Health Services Superanuation Division,
   DSS, Hesketh House, Fleetwood, Lancashire FY7 8LG.
DSS Health Services Superannuation,
   5a Frederick Street, Belfast BT1 2KW.
Scottish Office Superannuation Division,
   St Margaret's House, 151 London Road, Edinburgh EH8 7TG.

MEMBERSHIP OF TRADE UNIONS

Trade unions help with legal assistance, represent their members, offer negligence insurance cover, have benevolent funds and actively promote further education and training. These are just some of the reasons for joining a good trade union.

There is no obligation on the employer's part to recognize a trade union but in practice most employers have no objection to trade unions and appreciate the service they offer to employees. Most nurses are advised during their training to become members of a union for reasons of indemnity if nothing else. The main unions used by nurses are:

RCN (Royal College of Nursing)
POA (Prison Officers Association)
UNISON (the newly formed union from NALGO, COHSE and NUPE)
NALGO (National and Local Government Officers Association)
COHSE (Confederation of Health Service Employees)
NUPE (National Union of Public Employees)

There are different reasons for joining each of these unions. Details of the unions, what they have to offer members and their policies can be obtained from the local stewards or the headquarters.

USEFUL READING

McMullen J (1984) *Rights at Work – a Guide to Employment Law*. London: Pluto Press.

USEFUL ADDRESSES

Confederation of Health Service Employees,
    Glen House, High Street, Banstead, Surrey SM7 2LH.
National and Local Government Officers Association,
    1 Mabledon Place, London WC1H 9AJ.
National Union of Public Employees,
    Civic House, 20 Grand Depot Road, Woolwich, London SE18 6SF.
Prison Officers Association,
    Cronin House, 245 Church Street, Edmonton, London N9 9HW.
Royal College of Nursing,
    20 Cavendish Square, London W1M 0AB.

LEGAL ASPECTS OF NURSING

Legal aspects of nursing are a study in their own right. Lawyers are actively involved in the handling of an increasing number of medical negligence cases each year.

Aspects of civil law which may particularly affect nurses are trespass and negligence, negligence being the most common either against nurses or in medical cases in which nurses are involved.

To bring a case based on negligence the aggrieved party must be able to prove that a duty of care was owed to them, that this duty was breached and that as a result they sustained damage. Trespass against the person includes issues such as restraint of patients.

With the increasing pace of change in nursing, fluctuation in staffing levels, increased complexity of care and treatment, along with greater specialization, nurses need to be very aware of legal obligations to clients, relatives, colleagues, the scope of professional practice and the organization within which they work. Attendance on a study day or some further reading on this subject would be prudent.

PROFESSIONAL CODE OF CONDUCT

The United Kingdom Central Council for Nurses, Midwives and Health Visitors is the legal professional body with the remit and power to decide, define and monitor rules, regulations and standards. For this purpose the UKCC has produced the *Code of Professional Conduct* (UKCC 1992) which applies to all nurses, midwives and health visitors. A copy of this may be obtained from the UKCC. Breach of the code can result in disciplinary action by the UKCC and may lead to the offending nurse, midwife or health visitor being removed from the Register of Practitioners. Disciplinary hearings are held in different parts of the country and as part of the profession's practice can be attended by those nurses, midwives or health visitors who wish to observe a hearing. A list of dates and venues of hearings is published by the UKCC and can be obtained from the Central Office.

Exercising Accountability and *The Scope of Professional Practice* (UKCC 1992) are essential reading. The increased specialization within branches of nursing, more sophisticated techniques and practices have led to extension of the traditional nurse's role. The UKCC policy decision is that certification of extended role tasks limits the scope of practice and that a more flexible approach within the code of conduct is required. This is particularly important for senior nurses defining and implementing policies and practice. It is equally significant for the nurse, midwife or health visitor wishing to extend their role.

Leaflets which discuss the rulings within the *Code of Conduct* in more depth can be obtained from the UKCC.

REFERENCES

UKCC (1992) *Code of Professional Conduct.* London: UKCC.
UKCC (1992) *The Scope of Professional Practice.* London: UKCC.
UKCC (1992) *Exercising Accountability.* London: UKCC.

USEFUL READING

Bayliss P F (1987) *The Law Relating to Health Care Professions.* Beckenham: Ravenswood Publications.
Burnard P & Chapman C (1993) *Professional and Ethical Issues in Nursing,* 2nd edn. London: Scutari Press.
Dimond B (1990) *Legal Aspects of Nursing.* Hemel Hempstead: Prentice Hall.
Hargreaves M (1979) *Practical Law for Nurses.* Tunbridge Wells: Pitman Medical Publishing.
Young A P (1981) *Legal Problems in Nursing Practice.* London: Harper and Row Ltd.
Young A P (1993) *Law and Professional Conduct in Nursing,* 2nd edn. London: Scutari Press.

CAREER BREAKS

Current trends within both the nursing profession and employment generally would suggest that periods of employment are likely to be shorter and more intense with breaks in between. These breaks may occur as a result of personal circumstances such as pregnancy or may be enforced by burnout symptoms or redundancy. Some people may simply require a new challenge, change or temporary reduction in workload. An acceptance, based upon the Department of Health's workforce survey (1991), that the nursing population no longer pursues a full-time traditional career from qualification to retirement, is beginning to re-shape attitudes towards career breaks and employees. Employers are beginning to recognize experience gained outside nursing which can contribute to nursing in new ways. Multi-skilling is now a desirable quality in the qualified practitioner.

Individuals who approach career development outside nursing as a positive step towards becoming a multi-skilled professional and who can contribute to nursing with added qualities in the future may have a much greater chance of continued employment and stimulating experiences throughout their life.

Career breaks are not a concept or reality that seems to fit into the nursing profession with ease. Traditional career routes from basic training were seen as a slow progression through the ranks without a career break. Individuals who left the profession for many reasons found and still find it very difficult to return in any other capacity than basic grade nurses. Return to nursing is an issue addressed by PREP but the main emphasis is upon updating the individual at the point of re-entry. The level at which a nurse can re-enter the profession after an absence does seem to be a matter for ongoing debate at the moment and is most likely to be an issue that will be decided between the employer and individual nurse themselves.

The purpose of this section is not to discuss the problems of re-entry into the profession but to concentrate upon career breaks as a positive event. Properly planned career breaks rather than hasty exit could have considerable benefits with minimal problems upon re-entry into nursing. Career breaks are different for each individual and are taken for many reasons, with or without the intention to return to nursing.

Albeit at a slow pace, the profession is at last beginning to look at attracting nurses back into the profession, not least because of the considerable expense involved in training and recruitment. Nurses considering a career break should therefore plan their career break effectively so that the path back into nursing will be easier.

Career breaks refresh nurses and enable them to gain other skills, recuperate, find new direction or re-enthuse them, all of this at no cost to the organization within which the nurse is currently employed. Nurses who have employers who may be able to offer them employment at a later date may find it helpful to discuss the subject. Managers who are looking to retain staff and cut down on recruitment expenditure and repeated induction programmes may be receptive to a nurse who intends to leave a job, but would prefer to have a career break or time out.

Since 'career breaks' in this context means leaving the paid employment of one employer for a new set of circumstances with or without the intention of returning later, clearly the nurse needs to plan the time on a number of levels.

An analysis of the reasons for leaving will give the individual a clearer picture of the type of experience that he/she should undertake during the career break. It will probably be useful to acquire some career advice and information about types of potential employment and contracts.

Voluntary service abroad, undertaking a part-time qualification in psychology or accountancy are all useful and it could be relevant to discuss how they would fit into your professional portfolio. The number of opportunities and variety are enormous; sometimes, therefore, it is difficult for any employer to establish the relevance and worth of the experience. Make it easier for any potential employer to assess the experience and its relevance to them. Keep records of your activities during the career break and particularly note any new skills. How relevant are these skills to nursing? Which skills are particularly relevant and how are they applicable? What will the new skills contribute to nursing and to the particular ward or unit? Match up the skills and experience gained during the career break and credit them towards the nursing professional situation. Be able to justify their relevance to potential employers.

The point of re-entry into nursing will be different for each individual and will depend upon available vacancies. A properly planned income during the career break period should enable the nurse to wait for the right opportunity and status.

Unplanned career breaks can be used as equally valid time and experiences can be counted towards re-entry. The nurse needs to assess the experience with hindsight and its relevance to the new nursing post.

The importance and relevance of maintaining a professional profile during a career break from nursing cannot be emphasized enough. The direct evidence of other skills and education gained can be extremely useful when applying to return to nursing. The profile itself may contain evidence that will be useful within an organization that uses a credit accumulation and transfer scheme or accreditation of prior learning as part of its development programme. In many instances skills and sometimes qualifications are transferable; this is discussed in more depth in Section Two of this volume and in the training and education part of Section Three.

There are a tremendous number of opportunities outside nursing which may be of interest to nurses. This volume concentrates on career opportunities that are allied to nursing or are useful with nursing qualifications.

REFERENCES

Department of Health (1991) *NHS Workforce in England: Executive Summary.* London: DoH.

USEFUL READING

Davis C (1990) *The Collapse of the Conventional Career: the Future of Work and its Relevance for Post Registration Education in Nursing.* Sheffield: ENB Publications.

McSweeney P (1991) The collapse of the conventional career. *Nursing
 ' Times*, **87**(31): 26–8.
Schroeder I (1991) Different paths. *Nursing Times*, **87**(31): 31–2.
Willis J (1991) Equal to the task. *Nursing Times*, **87**(31): 29–30.

5

Analysing your Career Position and Deciding Direction

A new opportunity requires careful planning if the opportunity is going to mean more than simply escape from the present situation; the new direction should be a window of opportunity that enhances your working life. This opportunity should build upon your hopes, values and skills, developing you as an individual and in the process contributing to society in general.

For many individuals the way forward is not always apparent. Lack of confidence, personal constraints and limited access to information all add to the difficulty of deciding direction. Even for those who have a clear picture of their future, the pathway may not always be as planned and goals may have to be changed. Both the professional and career opportunities that are available to nurses are increasing rapidly as nursing becomes more specialized, and outside the profession it is becoming easier to access other training and employment using the growing number of transferable qualifications that are now available.

The starting point for anybody who is contemplating a new approach to their working life has to be a greater understanding of their circumstances, personal constraints, skills and achievements. This volume cannot give you that understanding but it aims to help highlight some of the areas to consider and outlines a simple self-analysis process that could be undertaken each time a new challenge is anticipated. Personal needs must be met and personal qualities have to be right for the opportunity if it is to remain an opportunity and not become an encumbrance. The nurse who has not considered the intellectual requirements of a course or its long-term funding is unlikely to be able to complete the course. The individual who takes a job away from home because it is a good opportunity, but the travelling is too much, is unlikely to stay very long, or will have to change personal circumstances to meet the new job. Maslow (1954) identifies the hierarchy of human needs from basic physiological needs through to intellectual self-actualization. Successfully identifying your basic needs and meeting them is likely to provide a firmer foundation for advancement. This, combined with some indication of the key things that are important to you in the new opportunity, will begin to provide some clues to the way forward.

Some general tips:

- decide the time-frame within which you want to achieve your goals;
- set realistic goals;
- ask friends to help in the profiling stage;
- be realistic about the opportunity – a quiet person who enjoys working closely in a team is unlikely to make a good sales- person;
- when you have found the opportunity, work at it;
- build upon your strengths;
- try to conquer your weaknesses;
- make use of all the careers advisory services that you can find to help you make your decision;
- make use of a professional careers analysis service;
- undertake self-analysis.

SELF-ANALYSIS TOOL

The following self-analysis tool has been included as a rough guide only. For those who would like a much more in-depth analysis, a detailed personality and career analysis is available from professional career consultants. A good analysis is money well invested. It will help you to identify your own situation and the types of opportunities that are open to you in much more depth. However, these can be costly and identifying a reputable consultant is not always easy.

Work through the sections identifying those particular qualities that apply to you. Make a list of these qualities and use it to match up against job descriptions, career and professional opportunities. The word 'opportunities' could be applied equally to the nurse who is happy in his/her working situation with no desire to leave to the nurse who is contemplating leaving the profession.

The self-analysis process outlined is divided into six sections.

Section A assesses reasons for other opportunities and highlights issues that you will want to consider in a new opportunity; section B looks at commitment; section C considers you in your current workplace; section D considers constraints; section E examines motives; section F looks at personality issues.

A   Reasons for looking for other opportunities

Promotion
Stimulation
Money
Tired of your current job
A new direction
Other – state
What is wrong with your current job?
What is right with your current job?
What do you enjoy most about your current job?
What do you find hardest to do in your current job?

B   Your commitment to new opportunities

Time you are prepared to commit to the opportunity.
Finance you are prepared to commit.
How committed:
  Very
  Partially
  Mildly

C   Qualities that describe you in the workplace

Practical
Theoretical
Team leader
Team member
Like responsibility
Not keen on responsibility
Enjoy the challenge of change
Dislike too much change
Like working on your own
Do not like working on your own
Can motivate yourself
Need others to help motivate you
Assertive
Not very assertive
Cope with stress well
Cannot cope with stress well
Other – state

D Constraints

Yes/No   1–10

Time
Money
Family/people
Housing

(Decide how much of a constraint each item is to you on a scale of one to ten.)

E What is important to you in a new job?

Security
Promotion
Better working hours/flexibility
Independence
Support
Clinical
Teaching/education
Management
Nursing
Other

F Your personality

Easy-going	Responsible
Practical	Anxious
Adaptable	Shy
Intellectual	Punctual
Relaxed	Tolerant
Generous	Popular
Extrovert	Ambitious
Understanding	Hardworking
Confident	Quick
Persevering	Well organized
Reliable	Flair
Cooperative	Noisy
Cheerful	Competetive
Thoughtful	Modest
Sensitive	Aggressive
Sociable	Lacking in confidence

Tidy	Energetic
Untidy	Considerate
Moody	Humorous
Honest	Patient

Upon completion of the self-analysis tool a clearer picture of the reasons for a new opportunity, the commitment to it and constraints should have emerged.

REFERENCE

Maslow A H (1954) *Motivation and Personality.* New York: Harper.

USEFUL READING

Bayley J (1990) *How to Get a Job After 45.* London: Kogan Page.
Burston D (ed) (1991) *A–Z of Careers and Jobs.* London: Kogan Page.
Godfrey G & Plumbley P (1988) *Changing Your Job After 35.* London: Kogan Page.
Humphries J 1986 *Part-time Work.* London: Kogan Page.
JIIG-CAL (1991) *Job File 91.* London: Headway.
Schober J (1989) Making a job change. *Nursing Times,* **85**(22): 33–4.

USEFUL ADDRESSES

Career Analysts,
  Career House, 90 Gloucester Place, London W1H 4BL.
Centre for Professional Employment Counselling,
  Sundridge Park Management Centre, Plaistow Lane, Bromley, Kent BR1 3JW.
Careers Research and Advisory Centre,
  Sheraton House, Castle Park, Cambridge CB3 0AX.
Institute of Careers Officers,
  27a Lower High Street, Stourbridge, West Midlands DY8 8AB.

Section Two

The Opportunities

1

Return to Nursing

For any nurse who leaves either the profession or a particular branch of the profession and then wishes to return the experience can be intimidating. Feelings of incompetence, isolation and lack of confidence are often expressed. Professional skills appear to decline during absence from the profession but are quickly regained after a period of re-training. Many nurses find that professional issues have undergone tremendous amounts of change and that practical aspects of nursing have become much more sophisticated.

The profession itself is becoming more aware of the issues surrounding re-entry and the conditions of re-entry. Most nurses coming back into nursing or changing from one branch to another experience a loss of status. Ward sisters return as junior staff nurses, senior nurses find it difficult to find posts that attract them. This is slowly changing.

For the qualified nurse returning to practice after a career break or experience in a different branch of nursing the problems are just the same. In an attempt to rectify the situation the United Kingdom Central Council published a proposal in its Post Registration Education and Practice project which recommended that all nurses returning to practice with less than 100 days or 750 hours of nursing experience in the preceding five years should undertake a Return to Practice course before being placed on the register. The Central Council suggests that Return to Practice courses must meet the UKCC's requirements and be approved by a National Board.

BACK TO NURSING COURSES

The English, Scottish and Welsh National Boards currently run a number of approved Return to Practice courses. Course Number 902 Return to Nursing is approved by the English National Board. Full

29

details of these courses can be obtained from the National Board's Careers Advisory Services.

For any nurse considering leaving or returning to the profession, an active plan to maintain professional competence is required. There are a number of ways of preparing for return into the profession.

CONFERENCES AND STUDY DAYS

If you hope to return to work in a specialty, this is a particularly good way of updating yourself on current issues. Invariably there are trade exhibitors at these events who will be demonstrating equipment, treatments and other items of current value, and invariably one makes valuable contacts at conferences and study days; contacts with whom you can keep in touch and ask for further information. Many conferences have packages of material which include valuable references to literature, products and practitioners.

Conferences and study days are advertised within special interest groups and in the nursing press. *Nursing Times* and *Nursing Standard* have frequent advertisements for interesting and relevant study days.

Choose study days that are run by well-known institutions with credible speakers. Ascertain before you go if there will be a letter of attendance upon completion of the day. Keep a record of each session's contents and duration. Gain credit points for study undertaken whenever possible. Contact your local college of nursing for local courses.

VOLUNTARY WORK

Most hospitals, care homes and other major organizations have voluntary helpers in various capacities. An ideal way of getting back into the environment without being clinically involved is to volunteer for work in an appropriate setting. Quite apart from the obvious benefits, sometimes personal contact with the right people can help you to get the next job in nursing.

The National Council of Voluntary Services (NCVS) acts as an umbrella service for voluntary organizations. At a local level the NCVS have as part of their function volunteer bureaux which act as job centres for voluntary workers. Notice of vacancies or needs are sent from organizations, such as conservation groups and Help the Aged, to the bureaux. If you are contemplating voluntary work, contact your local National Council for Voluntary Services who are usually listed in the telephone directory; alternatively, approach the National Council for the address of your local council.

If you know the organization within which you wish to work, approach the voluntary services manager. Many major organizations have designated managers.

The Volunteer Centre UK is another national organization of interest to voluntary workers. The volunteer centre offers information, advice and support to volunteers themselves. This organization is linked to the pages available at the weekend on CEEFAX teletext, which provides a section for the voluntary services.

READING AND LITERATURE

Good nursing journals such as *Nursing Standard* and *Nursing Times* have current issues as headline items. Keep a list of all the articles and books that you read. Should you wish to refer to them again they will be easier to find and a comprehensive up-to-date bibliography could be useful if you decide to undertake further studies.

OPEN AND DISTANCE LEARNING

An increasing number of agencies offer information about open and distance learning courses. To name but a few, the Open University, the Open College and the South Bank University all have information about a variety of courses. The English National Board Careers Advisory Service has a database from which you can obtain computer printouts of courses available throughout the United Kingdom, addresses and course content details. Since there are more than 500 courses on the database, it is helpful to be specific about the subjects you are interested in when you contact the service.

Open and distance learning both require a great deal of commitment from the student. Before you undertake this method of study it is useful to identify the time and resources that will be required. Most open and distance learning projects offer some form of support, and in some cases group work, so that the experience need not be an isolated one.

BEFORE RETURNING TO PRACTICE

Given the current PREP requirements and the feelings of most nurses returning to work or changing from one branch to another, it is essential to find an employer who will offer you not only an induction programme but a proper back to nursing course. Before you commence in the new employment, find time to discuss your specific development needs with your immediate employer. An action plan that identifies your strengths and weaknesses could save much embarrassment and help you become more confident and regain skills more quickly. If at all possible speak to a nurse who has returned to nursing and undertaken a return to practice course. Colleges running the ENB 902 Return to Practice courses may be able to help you find a contact. If possible enrol for an ENB 902 course.

REFERENCES

United Kingdom Central Council (1991) *Post Registration Education and Practice Proposals.* London: UKCC.

USEFUL READING

Heywood-Jones I (1990) *Back to Nursing with Confidence.* Oxford: Heinemann Medical.
Laurent C (1989) Born again nurses. *Nursing Times,* **85**(23): 46–8.
Morton-Cooper A (1989) *Return to Nursing – a Guide for Nurses and Health Visitors.* Basingstoke: Macmillan Education.

USEFUL ADDRESSES

National Council for Vocational Qualifications,
   Information Service, 222 Euston Road, London NW1 2BZ.
National Council for Voluntary Organisations,
   26 Bedford Square, London WC1B 3HV.
Open College,
   Suite 470, St James Buildings, Oxford Street, Manchester M1 6FQ.
Open University,
   PO Box 48, Milton Keynes MK7 6AB.
Volunteer Centre UK,
   29 Lower Kings Road, Berkhamsted, Hertfordshire HP4 2AB.

2

Community, Midwifery and Paediatric Nursing

DISTRICT NURSING

District nurses work as part of a team which is attached to a local general practitioner's clinic. Each of the nurses have their own caseload and are responsible for assessing, planning and implementing the care in accordance with the rest of the health care team. In practice the district nurse is much more than a visiting nurse. He/she is often seen as friend and counsellor who is directly responsible for nursing care and patient education.

District nurses have a diverse and challenging role that has to overcome class, language and culture barriers. The district nurse may have patients in care homes, the patient's own home or may see patients in the doctor's surgery.

The district nurse is a guest in the patient's home and has to work in conditions that can range from glamorous to unsanitary. Unsocial hours and different weather conditions are as much a part of the job as is the tremendous job satisfaction that comes from delivering personal care. District nurses often gain much of their job satisfaction from the independence that they enjoy and the close patient contact.

Training for the District Diploma includes academic study in a higher education institution together with a period of supervised practice.

Information about courses available locally can be obtained from the National Boards of Nursing, Midwifery and Health Visiting or from the local District Health Authority.

District nurses can develop their careers by moving on to a senior nurse position which may be either management or a clinical nurse specialist, such as MacMillan nurse or diabetes specialist. District nurse recordable qualifications enable the holder to achieve the equivalent of specialist level within PREP.

OCCUPATIONAL HEALTH NURSING

Qualification for the role of occupational health nurse is the Diploma in Occupational Health. Qualifications required by nurses wanting to undertake the training include registered nurse status and evidence of recent study plus an evident interest in occupational health and an understanding of the role. Courses are usually at institutions of higher education. Some open learning occupational health courses are planned.

Employment is available within industry, the health services, commerce and education. Occupational nurses may be employed as independent practitioners within an organization, usually attached to a personnel department, or may be part of a large department of occupational health nurses working within a water authority, for example.

The emphasis of occupational health nursing is upon prevention of health problems and promotion of healthy living and working conditions. There is a small amount of basic first aid and screening attached to this role. Much of the occupational health nurse's goals are achieved by monitoring the workforce and workplace, combined with education and training programmes.

The challenge of occupational health nursing lies within changing attitudes and improving conditions. The occupational health nurse may also be a counsellor and friend for employees.

Some nurses that do not have the certificate may be employed by organizations, although increasingly employers require nurses to have the certificate before commencing the job.

Scutari Press has produced an occupational health nurse's development profile in cooperation with the Royal College of Nursing Special Interest Group. Open learning materials for the occupational health nurse include assessment packages.

MIDWIFERY

Midwifery training is currently of 18 months duration, based at a teaching hospital and attached to a college of nursing. The midwife works as a member of the multi-disciplinary team caring for prospective parents during the antenatal period and up to 28 days after the birth of the baby. Many midwifery units are trying to maintain continuity of care and allocate to each mother a midwife who is responsible for her care throughout pregnancy and after the birth. Traditionally, midwives rotate through the labour ward, antenatal and postnatal wards and clinics with time also spent in the community. Midwives have to undertake a statutory periodic update in order to be able to continue to practise. Midwives have, in effect, an extended role and are independent practitioners in their own right. Some midwives have broken away from the traditional centres of employment and set up in private practice in order to give a much more personal service to a few families. Working with families at a particularly emotional point in family life, midwives provide a sensitive and caring service that is often remembered by the family for years.

Some midwives choose to undertake the advanced diploma in midwifery, move into management or become a senior clinical nurse. Full details of the training and course availability can be obtained from the National Board of Nursing, Midwifery and Health Visiting. The Distance Learning Centre of the South Bank University has produced an open learning midwifery update.

HEALTH VISITOR

Health visitors take over the care of newborn babies at the age of 28 days; the family of young children and the children themselves are the primary responsibility of the health visitor. Development progress monitoring and access to various health services are provided by the health visitor.

Health visitors are attached to a general practitioner's clinic and work as part of the health care team providing community-based health promotion education and advice. The role of health visitor is an independent one, with a caseload which reflects local conditions and requirements. As counsellor and friend, the health visitor supports both the practical and psychological needs of clients. Typical activities can include teaching a mother how to choose and prepare healthy foods for her young family, or assessing a child's development progress and special needs. The ability to be sensitive to situations and individuals is essential in this role.

Training is undertaken at higher education institutions and is open to registered nurse status nurses who are also registered midwives or have undertaken a short course in midwifery. Health visitor training courses can be taken in a number of ways.

Placement is usually by secondment and may by arrangement be an extended course to take account of personal circumstances.

Further details can be obtained from the National Boards of Nursing, Midwifery and Health Visiting.

SCHOOL NURSE

The school nurse has a special remit to promote health and wellbeing in the population of school children. Visiting the school to immunize

and check children generally, the school nurse is well placed to identify children at risk and other problems, such as infestation.

School nurses may take part in the general programme and deliver
educational sessions on health-related issues. Working closely with the
teaching staff, school nurses have a unique and rewarding role. School
nursing can be an attractive option for the nurse who has family commitments of his or her own.

Nurses wishing to become school nurses must undergo a 12-week
training programme leading to a statement of attendance. Half the
course is theory and half is supervised practice. Applicants for the
course are usually seconded by their employer.

PRACTICE NURSE

Practice nurses are attached to doctors' surgeries and have varying
degrees of responsibilities. Some nurses complement the doctor's work
by giving immunizations, carrying out other practical procedures and
influencing clients to think about their own health. Others have a much
more independent role and are virtually practitioners in their own right.
The content of the role varies from practice to practice. Health education and promotion are a major part of the practice nurse's role.
The practice nurse has to be extremely skilful and competent in order
to use the small amount of time with each client to the full. Clinics
such as the 'well woman clinic' and diabetic clinics are organized by
the practice nurse.

While there are no obligatory qualifications beyond basic training, in
reality most nurses now undertake the English National Board Practice
Nurse Course. The course lasts for ten days and successful students
are awarded a statement of attendance.

The Royal College of Nursing has a special interest group for practice
nurses who have produced a practice nurse profile, available from
Scutari Press.

A list of institutions offering the practice nurse course can be obtained
from the National Boards of Nursing, Midwifery and Health Visiting. A
number of further education colleges now run various courses which are
relevant to the practice nurse and include subjects such as computing
for health care workers.

NURSE PRACTITIONERS

A small group of nurses who work from and in doctors' surgeries
with an extended role, nurse practitioners undertake diagnostic work
and prescribe care independently of doctors but in cooperation with

them. The Royal College of Nursing Institute of Advanced Nurse Education currently offers a two-year part-time diploma course for nurse practitioners.

NURSE TUTORS

Nurse tutors occupy a number of positions in the nursing profession and can now be found not only in colleges of nursing but also working independently for organizations such as *Nursing Times* Open Learning.

The role is an extremely rewarding one, which acts as both an educator and mentor to students. The nurse tutor is also a friend and counsellor. Nurse tutors may choose to specialize in either post-basic or basic training, concentrating on a particular interest, such as community care.

Some nurse tutors are purely academic and are based in colleges of nursing, while others have some elements of practice included in their work. Most nurse tutors are responsible for a group of students. A good subject knowledge, patience and an academic inclination are essential for this type of job. Nurse education has moved away from the more formal style of teaching to a student-centred, self-directed learning mode. Assignments, research and learning contracts are all activities that are coordinated and facilitated by the nurse tutor, but not directed by them. The relative explosion in nursing literature and research that is available to the student requires the tutor to update continually and to have read widely around the subject.

Nurse education is rapidly becoming a graduate status profession; many nurse tutors are undertaking research and publishing articles while completing a degree course. PREP indicates that all tutors/teachers should be graduates, have an advanced qualification and an appropriate teaching qualification.

Currently, nurses wishing to undertake tutor training must have at least three years' recent clinical experience in an approved area and additional certificated professional development in addition to registered nurse status. Courses are undertaken at higher education establishments and are usually undertaken on a full-time secondment basis.

Tutors of midwifery require at least 12 months' practice as registered midwives prior to commencement of training. The course is full-time by secondment and is undertaken at an institute of higher education. Similarly, the nurse tutor in health visiting or district nursing requires the relevant professional qualifications and at least three years' experience as a district nurse or health visitor.

Nurses wishing to become teachers or tutors could undertake courses such as ENB 998/997 Teaching and Assessing or City and Guilds 730.

The traditional tutor courses are gradually being replaced by approved degree courses.

FAMILY PLANNING NURSE

Health education is a key responsibility of this role, as is a mature approach to personal problems. The family planning nurse has an independent role which is linked into the community services. Operating through general practitioner clinics or family planning centres the nurse deals with a variety of problems from counselling to contraception. Assessment, planning and implementation of a personal programme for each client is part of this demanding role. Sometimes other problems present themselves during consultation and the nurse needs to refer the client to an appropriate source of help. The family planning nurse also has a commitment to education and may be included in part of a local school's education programme for adult life.

Not all pregnancies are planned and some aspects of the family planning nurse's role concern sensitive issues such as termination of pregnancy or support for the single mother. Much support, advice and counselling are needed in these circumstances.

The family planning service makes a major contribution to society and the nurse's role within the occupation is both rewarding for the individual and essential to society. Family planning nurses are registered general nurses, midwives or health visitors.

REGISTERED SICK CHILDREN'S NURSE

Central to the welfare of the child is the family's wellbeing; a children's nurse cares for the whole family when a child is admitted into the hands of health care staff.

Sick children's nursing embraces a large number of conditions, since children are cared for together in hospitals because of their age and development needs rather than their clinical complaint. In a children's ward the qualified nurse may have to work with children of all ages and degrees of ill health.

Most children's wards have a school attached to them or some form of education programme and teacher. Paediatric units aim to disrupt the child's life, relationships, education and development as little as possible.

Many children's nurses have a particular affinity for children and are able to communicate with them at an appropriate level, gaining the child's trust and cooperation.

Registered general nurses, registered mental nurses and registered mental handicap nurses can undertake further training to become a children's nurse. The registered general nurse training is a 53-week course (in the case of those with extensive experience the course is 26 weeks). Registered mental and mental handicap nurses can undertake a 73-week course. Further details of the courses and training establishments are available from the National Boards for Nursing, Midwifery and Health Visiting.

The National Boards offer a larger number of specialist courses for the nurse working with sick children. Courses range from the post-basic course in paediatric medical and surgical cardiothoracic nursing to nursing disturbed children and adolescents.

USEFUL READING

Bolden K & Tackle B (1984) *Practice Nurse Handbook.* Oxford: Blackwell.
Hopson B & Scally M (1981) *Lifeskills Teaching.* London: McGraw-Hill.
Kenworthy N & Nicklin P (1989) *Teaching and Assessing in Nursing Practice: an Experiential Approach.* London: Scutari Press.
Luker K & Orr J (1985) *Health Visiting.* Oxford: Blackwell.
Readman U (1991) *Standards of Care: School Nursing.* London: Scutari Press.
Robertson C (1988) *Health Visiting in Practice.* Edinburgh: Churchill Livingstone.
Walkin L (1990) *Teaching and Learning in Further and Adult Education.* Cheltenham: Thornes.
White Paper (1989) *Caring for People: Community Care in the Next Decade and Beyond.* London: HMSO.
Wreford B M (1992) *Environmental Assessment of the Workplace.* London: Scutari Press.
Wroe J B (ed) (1993) *Handbook of Community Nursing.* Chichester: Media Medica.

USEFUL JOURNALS

Community View, Smith and Nephew, Hull.
Health Visitor, Health Visitors' Association, BMA.
Journal of District Nursing, PTM Publishing, Sutton.
Midwife and Health Visitor, Newbourne Health Services, London.
Midwives' Chronicle, Nursing Notes Ltd, London.
Midwifery, Churchill Livingstone, Edinburgh.
Nurse Education Today, Churchill Livingstone, Edinburgh.
Occupational Health, Aldwych Publishing, London.
Occupational Health Review, Eclipse, London.

Paediatric Nursing, Nursing Standard Publications, Harrow.
Practice Nurse, Reed Healthcare Communications, Sutton.
Practice Nursing, Mark Allen Publishing, London.
Primary Health Care, Nursing Standard Publications, Harrow.
Professional Care of Mother and Child, Media Medica Publications Ltd,
   Chichester.

USEFUL ADDRESSES

Association of Paediatric Nurses,
   c/o Central Nursing Office, Hospital for Sick Children, Great Ormond
   Street, London WC1N 3JH.
Association of Radical Midwives,
   62 Greetby Hill, Ormskirk, Lancs L39 2DT.
Distance Learning Centre,
   South Bank University, South Bank Technopark, 90 London Road,
   London SE1 6LN.
District Nursing Association,
   57 Lower Belgrave Street, London SW1 0LR.
Health Visitors' Association,
   50 Southwark Street, London SE1 1UN.
Occupational Health Nurses' Association,
   c/o Royal College of Nursing, 20 Cavendish Square, London
   W1M 0AB.
Royal College of Midwives,
   15 Mansfield Street, London W1M 0BE.

3

Nursing in the Specialties

FURTHER STATUTORY TRAINING

Further statutory training is, for some people, a means of changing to a different type of nursing, increasing knowledge or achieving promotion.

Registered general nurses can become registered sick children's nurses, registered mental nurses and registered nurses mental health. The registered sick children's nurse can convert to registered general nurse, mental nurse and registered nurse mental health.

Nurses that have undertaken the registered mental nurse training can convert to registered general nurse and registered nurse mental health.

Finally, the registered nurse mental health can undertake general nurse training and mental nurse training.

The courses take between twelve and eighteen months. Full details of the colleges offering these courses and further details of course length and content can be obtained from the National Boards of Nursing, Midwifery and Health Visiting.

CLINICAL SPECIALIST COURSES

Clinical specialist courses run by the National Boards fall into two groups; some courses are certificated and the others are awarded statements of attendance. The category that a course falls into is decided by its content and length. A full list of courses that are currently being provided by colleges can be obtained from the National Boards. The variety is enormous and includes subjects such as renal nursing, accident and emergency nursing, stoma care, orthopaedic nursing and counselling.

In addition to full-length recordable and certificated courses there is a number of short courses and non-recordable qualifications. The courses are of differing lengths and involve clinical placements and theory blocks. The clinical placements are usually carried out under the guidance of mentors and supervisors. The theory blocks are under the supervision of nurse tutors with extensive experience and further qualifications in the relevant field. Considerable emphasis is placed upon self-directed learning under supervision. Learning contracts and agreements are drawn up between the college student and clinical area to enable this process to be safe and educationally valid, but not stifling.

Courses are often very popular and applicants should consider asking for secondment and applying for a place well in advance of the date that they would like to start. Some colleges are now accepting fee-paying students who have not been seconded. It may be easier to be offered a placement on courses that are under-subscribed if you have found your own funding. Further details of funding and finance can be found at the end of this volume.

Evidence of further study and preferably some project or research work is usually expected by the college interviewing applicants for advanced courses. A number of the National Board courses now attract credit accumulation and transfer ratings. Further details about the specific rating for each course can be obtained from the National Boards' Careers Services.

STUDY DAYS

In addition to the large number of specialist courses, a number of institutions and organizations offer individual study days and sessions.

Departments of Nursing in universities and other higher education establishments are using their facilities to accommodate study days. Traditionally colleges of nursing have had continuing education and in-service training departments attached to them that offer similar study sessions. Since the publication of the Post Registration Education and Practice Report from the UKCC, most study days now have some form of attendance certificate. Study days and sessions that have a strong clinical emphasis may cover subjects such as pressure area care and pain control. Sessions such as this do not always merit a full course since the topic can usually be covered in a day. These sessions fill in gaps that are not covered by full courses run by the National Boards. Some nurses may choose to extend their knowledge by attending a series of relevant study days and building up their expertise on a modular basis.

Attendance on any study course should be utilized afterwards. Objectives for attending the course may help nurses to apply the knowledge upon their return to the workplace and reflect upon it afterwards. Employers are becoming less willing to release nurses on study sessions unless they apply the knowledge upon their return.

CONFERENCES AND CONVENTIONS

Conferences and conventions are particularly useful ways of extending clinical knowledge. Professional organizations such as the Infection Control Nurses Group and the Wound Care Society hold annual conferences which act as a forum for practitioners from considerable distances apart. The speakers and exhibitors have a wealth of different, current information for the visiting nurse. Recent research and developments are often some of the main themes of the day. Company representatives attending these conferences are able to apprise specialist nurses of new products and correct usage of existing items.

Perhaps the main benefit of conferences and conventions is the contact with other professionals. Much of the real learning is often done over coffee and lunch! Many new friendships are forged and the chance to visit other clinical areas can be arranged. One of the benefits of this informal aspect of conferences and conventions is the cross-fertilization of ideas that takes place. This cannot be measured, but it is common knowledge that people come back from these events with many new ideas, most of which have come from other delegates.

4

Conversion to First Level Nurse

Application, waiting for a place and actually undertaking the course can be an extremely time-consuming and frustrating experience. It is therefore worth planning your application. Consider the qualifications that you have, your motivation for undertaking the course, the waiting list of other applicants and the particular entry requirements for the local course. Plan your course of action accordingly. Places are relatively scarce and competition is fierce. In the future the conversion course will be based upon the P2000 training and will reflect the needs of the future workforce. It would be worthwhile asking if your local college is taking steps to gain approval or designing a new-style course and, if so, how long before the course commences, what will the entry requirements be and other relevant details. It may be prudent to wait for new-style courses but it is something of a gamble, since the way forward on this issue is not yet clear.

See a tutor about your local situation and your particular position. A list of colleges of nursing can be obtained from the *Nurse Central Clearing House Handbook* available in colleges of nursing libraries, or it can be purchased from the Central Clearing House in Bristol.

Examine your motive for conversion. Justification for conversion must be to continue as a practical nurse in the clinical sense or to continue to a nurse specialist/senior nurse role. Individuals who wish to pursue a management or educationalist line in a non-nursing capacity may be well advised to consider other routes through the system.

If you choose to convert from second level to first level nurse the path will not be easy, but the end result should be rewarding.

Between making the decision to convert and actually obtaining a place on the conversion course there may be a considerable waiting period. Use this time to your advantage. If you do not have the basic entry and local requirements the first and obvious step is to obtain these.

Often the requirements will contain not only formal academic qualifications but also evidence of recent study. For those applicants who have all the formal qualifications required this may be the opportunity to look at less traditional forms of study and to consider routes that may offer other options. One such option is the open learning route offered by the Open University: the courses on offer can be built up as credits towards certificates, diplomas and degrees. One such diploma (Diploma in Health and Social Welfare) would offer a second level nurse a credible qualification, evidence of recent study and detailed study of areas allied to nursing care. Should you change your mind about conversion to first level, qualifications such as the Diploma in Health and Social Services could give you access to another career. In addition to this, the Health and Social Welfare Course will give you two of the six credits needed to complete an Open University degree. Contact the Open University for further details.

Currently there are two methods of undertaking the conversion course from second to first level nurse. The traditional route is to obtain a place at a local college of nursing and undertake the course full time, usually with secondment from the workplace. For the second level nurse working in the private sector it is not so easy to secure a place on one of the courses.

The other method is the new Open Learning Conversion Course offered by *Nursing Times* with approval from the English National Board. To be able to undertake this course you need to ensure that you are able to find the study time and to gain the relevant practical experience. This course is a good option for second level nurses who are unable to undertake full-time training or who wish to pursue this line for other reasons.

Information about the above methods of conversion entry requirements and course details can be obtained from the *Nursing Times* Open Learning Centre and from your local college of nursing or the National Boards for Nursing and Midwifery.

Not all second level nurses will want to undertake the conversion or move into a different area of practice. Many may choose to remain within their current sphere of practice and look for opportunities that enable them to specialize and/or develop their current skills. Look for study sessions in the nursing press and consult the various professional bodies, for example the special interest groups run by organizations such as the Royal College of Nursing, The King's Fund Centre and colleges of nursing. It may be possible to contact second level nurses working in the same specialty in another part of the country and find out about courses on offer to them locally. Do not be afraid to ask your local Continuing Education Department to run something that may be appropriate. You may even wish to consider running your own study day or linking up with others to do so. Make sure you collect certificates/letters of attendance for all courses that you attend in preparation for future re-registration requirements.

For individuals who do not wish to convert but wish to broaden their horizons there are increasingly more opportunities for you to do so. BBC Television currently offers a number of open learning options for nursing which include the Open University programme of health-related issues and the *Nursing Standard*/RCN joint venture. In addition to this there are a large number of open learning opportunities available from other sources. Information about these courses can be obtained from the English National Board Database in Sheffield. You local college of health studies/nursing and further education colleges should have a number of options available. Information about courses on offer can be obtained from the college themselves, your local library or the local council's education department.

USEFUL READING

Laurent C (1989a) A private conversion. *Nursing Times*, **85**(42): 48–50.
Laurent C (1989b) Mass conversion. *Nursing Times*, **85**(29): 33–4.

USEFUL ADDRESSES

Nursing Standard Open Learning,
  Viking House, 17–19 Peterborough Road, Harrow, Middlesex HA1 2AX.
Nursing Times Open Learning,
  4 Little Essex Street, London WC2R 3LF.
Open University,
  PO Box 48, Milton Keynes MK7 6AB.

5

Opportunities for the Psychiatric Nurse

In addition to the vast number of opportunities available to nurses generally, as discussed elsewhere in this volume, psychiatric nurses have some choices that are particularly attractive and relevant.

COUNSELLING

Counselling courses of different types offer the qualified psychiatric nurse the chance to move into different types of employment. Specific organizations, such as charities and societies, employ individuals who have additional skills. Crisis, bereavement, rape and disturbed youth counselling are just some of the openings available. Social Services departments often have vacancies for trained counsellors. Behaviour modification counselling and support is required by organizations such as Alcoholics Anonymous and Health Authorities. Substance abuse is another specialist area within which the psychiatric trained nurse may choose to work.

The opportunities to develop individual relationships and to manage your own caseload are only some of the rewarding aspects of this type of role.

A number of National Board courses are particularly relevant to nurses who wish to gain further specialist skills. Contact the Careers Advisory Services of the National Boards for further details.

COMMUNITY PSYCHIATRIC NURSE

Community psychiatric nursing offers the challenge of caring for clients and their families within the home setting. Each community psychiatric nurse has their own caseload and works within a team of nurses covering a particular geographical area.

The rewards of helping an individual to lead life outside hospital and return to health in their own home cannot be underestimated. Much more emphasis is being placed upon nursing the psychiatric client within the community. The number of posts for psychiatric nurses in the community has increased over the last few years.

MANAGEMENT AND SENIOR NURSE POSTS

Nurse management and senior nurse posts are open to psychiatric nurses in a number of forms. Joint appointments such as clinical nurse managers and clinical nurse specialist offer the nurse employment at a higher level but still retaining some clinical input. Some management roles are purely administrative and are an excellent stepping stone into general management. A full discussion of the types of senior nurse roles appears elsewhere in this volume.

NURSE TUTOR/TEACHER

A number of psychiatric nurses progress to nurse education and specialize in different branches. Opportunities exist within basic and post-basic colleges of nursing. Some private health organizations employ the occasional psychiatric nurse tutor. Vacancies are usually advertised in the nursing press.

PRISON SERVICE AND FORENSIC PSYCHIATRY

In addition to the opportunities within the general prison hospitals and services, psychiatric nurses are employed to staff the specialist mental health units. Regional secure units housing particularly difficult clients have a constant need for psychiatric nurses with the right personal qualities to work in this sensitive environment.

OVERSEAS

The need for psychiatric nurses in other countries changes. Many nurses find it possible to gain employment in countries such as New Zealand and Australia, where their qualifications are accepted. Nurses wishing to work in Canada or the United States of America are subject to the same processes as the general nurse. See the chapter on working abroad for further details and addresses.

FURTHER STATUTORY TRAINING

Additional qualifications such as the registered general nurse certificate can be gained after undertaking a shortened training course. Further details of the length and type of training open to the psychiatric nurse can be found in this volume.

POST-BASIC COURSES

In addition to specific study days and courses there are a number of National Board courses that are relevant to the psychiatric nurse. These include topics such as psychiatric nursing within secure environments and the recognition and management of substance abuse. Many colleges now offer in-house training of different types for the post-basic student.

NURSE THERAPIST

The role of the nurse therapist is a relatively new one that looks as though it will continue to gain ground. The multi-skilling of nurses, in particular with therapy skills, is attractive to health care providers and satisfying for nurses themselves. Nursing can be successfully combined with a number of therapeutic activities such as massage and cognitive skills training.

National Board courses for psychiatric nurses

National Board courses for psychiatric nurses include the following:

Drug and alcohol dependency nursing.
Drug dependency nursing for nurses.
Adult behavioural psychotherapy.
Behaviour modification in mental handicap nursing.
Shared initiatives in residential and day services practice.
Rehabilitation of the mentally ill.
Developments in psychiatric nursing.
Care of the violent or potentially violent individual.
Principles of psychiatric nursing within secure environments. First level nurses.
Principles of psychiatric nursing within secure environments. Second level nurses.
Recognition and management of substance abuse.
Principles of psychosexual counselling.
Principles of community psychiatric nursing. Second level nurses.
Principles of community psychiatric nursing. First level nurses.
Care of people with mental illness in community residential and day services.

The above-mentioned are only some of the relevant courses. There are further courses that nurses working in the psychiatric branches of nursing may find useful. These include those courses that are allied to general nursing and other mental health care settings. Further details can be obtained from the Careers Advisory Services of the National Boards.

6

The Armed Forces

For the qualified nurse, the services offer some of the most secure and enjoyable opportunities currently available. The chance to work abroad with the forces is particularly attractive. All the services are keen to develop their nurses and in addition to a clearly defined professional structure offer a promotional structure within the service which is based upon the individual's performance. Length of service varies according to the particular force.

In general the entrance requirements are as follows:

- A clean bill of health, including good eyesight and certain height and weight restrictions.
- Current registration with the UKCC.
- Experience since qualifying is not always required.
- Certain nationality requirements.
- Successful completion of the normal application procedure and the particular force's basic training.
- The level at which a nurse enters the service will depend upon experience gained and the individual force itself.

Pay and conditions within the services are very favourable and include extra payment for certain duties, qualifications and postings. Board and lodgings for both single and married individuals are extremely reasonable. Postings abroad attract paid travel warrants for leave purposes up to four times a year. Serving employees are entitled to up to forty-five days' annual leave a year.

All the forces offer the qualified nurse the opportunity to apply for conversion to registered general nurse. It should be emphasized, however, that the services offer the opportunity to convert under the same conditions as the private and National Health Services – commitment to the service being a prime qualification for the candidate. Therefore the forces are unlikely to consider the second level nurse who wishes to enter solely to undertake the conversion course.

Most serving nurses gain their job satisfaction from the quality of the environment in which they work, excellent promotion prospects and the relatively high staff to patient ratio.

In return for a substantial investment in their workforce the forces expect a real commitment from serving individuals and loyalty to the force itself. Personal qualities, motivation, intelligence, application and ability coupled with a positive attitude are at least as important as the formal professional and academic qualifications.

Qualified nurses can enter into different branches within the forces and undertake other training, such as Radiography within the Royal Air Force. Each application will be considered on its own merits.

Qualified nurses who are interested in entering the forces should contact their nearest services careers offices for an informal discussion.

ROYAL AIR FORCE

(Princess Mary's Royal Air Force Nursing Service)

Opportunities for the first level nurse

First level nurses entering the Royal Air Force (RAF) can expect to enjoy some excellent working conditions and pay in return for hard work and commitment. The RAF is committed to developing and maintaining the highest standards of care. To this purpose it invests in its staff, often seconding individuals to undergo training.

Entry into the service can be either as a staff nurse or officer. Staff nurse status is open to first level general nurses immediately upon qualification. Applicants must pass the selection tests and an interview before admission into the service and should be between the ages of twenty-one and forty years.

Following a five-and-a-half-week training course for women or six weeks for men the new entrant is then posted to one of the RAF hospitals in the United Kingdom to begin their employment. The initial training is professional army training, and equips the new entrant for life within the RAF. It also marks the beginning of a career structure which runs parallel to that of the nursing role. Although classed as a non-combatant the RAF nurse has a professional commitment to the overall service and undertakes related tasks in addition to those required for the nursing role.

Promotion can be very rapid, rising through the ranks from Junior Technician to Flight Sergeant in less than four years. Promotion in the higher levels of the career structure is dependent upon the ability, effort and commitment of each individual.

New postings occur approximately every three years. This, combined with the excellent sporting and social facilities, helps to keep RAF nurses refreshed, fit and able to cope with new challenges.

Some nurses may be chosen or elect to apply for training as an inflight nurse. Aeromedical nursing has its own challenges. Each of the aeromedical nurses have two flight nursing attendants attached to them who assist with inflight duties of care. Promotion from staff nurse to nursing officer is based upon merit.

Direct entry officers are admitted as qualified registered nurses with at least one year's post-basic experience and a second professional qualification. Entry is between the ages of twenty-three and thirty-five years. Following a medical examination and interview the successful applicant undertakes the shortened specialist entry and re-entry course for officers. Officers can be admitted on short service commissions for four years, which may be extended for up to eight years. Alternatively, after an initial period of two years officers can apply for a permanent commission.

Nursing officers are admitted at the Flying Officer rank and progress upon merit and post availability to Group Captain. Entry can be above Flying Officer rank but this is dependent upon your experience within civilian health care and its relevance to the RAF's immediate needs.

The nursing officer role differs between war- and peacetime. During time of war the principal duties are to run services behind the front line. During peacetime the main duties are those of a leading clinician and manager.

In addition to the duties of nursing officer the role has a commitment to the RAF as a profession. Officers undertake duties related to general management in the centre in which they are based as part of the RAF officer's overall role.

The nursing officer has the opportunity to apply for secondment for further training that is relevant and to undertake specialist training such as that of aeromedical nursing.

OPPORTUNITIES FOR SECOND LEVEL NURSES

Second level nurses enter into the ranks within the technical services of the Medical Trade Group.

Applicants are interviewed by a Specialist Officer at Squadron Leader level who considers whether the applicant is suitable for service life, why the applicant wishes to be considered and if the application and candidate are good for the post. All applicants are shown around the RAF's extremely well-equipped hospitals and given an opportunity to consider the reality of life in the forces.

The policy of Princess Mary's Royal Air Force Nursing Service is to convert all its second level nurses to first level status in the course of time. To achieve this the RAF, who do not provide the conversion course training, have agreed a number of places on the NHS Hospital Conversion Courses.

Entry requirements are as follows. In addition to UKCC registration the candidate must be under forty years of age and have passed a few simple tests which will be offered at the local RAF Careers Information Office. Once selected by qualification, test, medical and interview procedures the successful candidate then undergoes a period of training. Six weeks of recruitment training at RAF Sanderby and sixteen days of Medical Trade Group basic course at RAF Halton are followed by posting to one of the RAF's hospitals in the UK at Halton or Wroughton.

Full details of the entry process, subsequent training and opportunities can be obtained from the local RAF careers service. A list of local RAF careers information offices is printed on the leaflet *PUB 413*, obtainable from the Director of Nursing Services (RAF) London.

ARMY

(Queen Alexandra's Royal Army Nursing Corps)

Opportunities for first level nurses

The Army nurse has the opportunity to work both abroad and at home in a variety of situations. Because of the nature of the service, serving nurses are perhaps more likely to see active service than the Royal Navy or Royal Air Force. The Army deploys nurses into a variety of situations on a regular basis.

The majority of first level general nurses enter into the Army as an officer after one year's post-basic experience. Nurses who have extensive experience can ask to have this taken into consideration; this could result in the new entrant being admitted to ranks as far as that of Captain.

Upon employment the new officer undertakes a field training programme with a high emphasis upon physical fitness and survival skills. Other training issues include responsibilities within the service and administration procedures. Individuals are then posted to their first hospital.

The Army places great emphasis upon its parallel career structure and actively encourages nurses to undertake further relevant study and promotion examinations. Further study such as specialist nursing courses can be applied for by serving nurses.

Nurses undertake contracts for short service commissions of two years, after which they can then apply for a transfer to a regular commission.

The Army offers excellent opportunities including rapid promotion, good salaries and conditions for those who are committed and prepared to work hard for the service.

Most serving nurses enjoy an exciting career with travel, new companions and new challenges regularly.

Opportunities for the second level nurse

Direct entry for the second level nurse is open to those nurses under the age of thirty-three years. The method of entry is by application, test and interview and a successful medical examination is essential. Most second level nurses are engaged on a three-year contract which can be renewed. All new entrants undergo a ten-week introductory training course at the QARANC training centre in Aldershot. Whether student, first or second level, each nurse has the initial ten-week training designed to give the new entrant details of military life, the organization and administration, and some basic fieldcraft. A very high emphasis is placed upon physical activities and physical fitness. QARANCs are encouraged to pursue their own favourite sports in addition to the regular exercise routines designed to help nurses cope in a variety of conditions. After the initial ten-week training direct entry second level nurses are sent to their first posting. As far as possible the Army tries to meet every nurse's preferred choice of posting.

In common with the other forces, the Army actively encourages nurses to undertake further training and study. The Army has its own training school and has a number of places for conversion from second level to first level nurse. The Army's conversion course is approved by the National Boards and applications are considered equally from both Army-trained and direct entry nurses. In addition to conversion the Army offers second level nurses the opportunity to undertake further specialist courses. These courses are usually undertaken at other centres outside the Army. The Army operates a system that allows it to add the length of attendance on the course (and therefore absence during secondment from the Army) to the period of enlistment.

In addition to advancement through the nursing career structure, the Army offers nurses the opportunity to progress on a different structure, the Army ranking system. Promotion through the ranks from Private can come very quickly and depends entirely upon the efforts of the individual.

In common with the other services, once enlisted it is not easy to move from one branch of the Army to another. If a second level nurse wishes to enter the Army in a different capacity the qualification will be considered in addition to the basic entry requirements for the specific field applied for. Other opportunities include: Dental Clerk Assistant,

Medical Clerk, Ward Stewardess, Laboratory Assistant, Pharmacy Technician and Radiographer.

For further details of nursing and nursing-related opportunities contact the QARANC Liaison Officer, Ministry of Defence.

ROYAL NAVY

(Queen Alexandra's Royal Navy Nursing Service)

OPPORTUNITIES FOR FIRST LEVEL NURSES

The Royal Navy Nursing Service offers some of the most exciting opportunities currently available to nurses. Work in the United Kingdom and abroad, as well as aboard ship, makes this one of the most challenging roles in nursing today. The Royal Navy (RN) encourages its nurses continuously to raise nursing care standards and to develop themselves professionally.

Entry can be as a direct entry first level general nurse or officer entry.

Direct entry first level nurses begin their career as staff nurses. Admission is by interview and medical. Successful applicants are then sent on an initial service training course. Applications are invited from first level general nurses aged twenty-one to twenty-eight years who have recently qualified having only limited or no post-basic experience.

Promotion within the ranks is upon merit and opportunity. After two years of service the RN staff nurse can apply to become an officer.

Close links are maintained between National Health Service training centres and the Royal Navy Service. Further study is actively encouraged particularly when it is directly relevant to service needs.

During peacetime postings are with hospitals in the United Kingdom and abroad. During time of war nurses are required to staff hospitals both on land and at sea in hospital ships. High emphasis is placed upon leading a balanced life. Sport and social activities are encouraged.

Direct entry officers undertake commissions on a short- or medium-term basis. Officers entering the service undertake a short orientation programme and then begin their service.

The role requires individuals to be leaders not only within nursing but also within the RN career structure. Officers undertake duties that are RN-related and often management-based. Although classed as a non-combatant serving officer the RN nursing officer can enjoy promotion within the RN career structure as well as the nursing profession.

Further details of direct entry for both staff nurses and officers can be obtained from the local Royal Navy Careers Office. The address should be available in the telephone directory or directly from Naval Headquarters.

OPPORTUNITIES FOR SECOND LEVEL NURSES

In common with the other forces entry follows from a successful written examination after which an interview and medical examination are held. After meeting the entry requirements and passing all the aforementioned examinations the candidate is required to attend a professional selection interview at the Royal Navy Hospital Haslar.

The first six weeks (female) and seven weeks (male) are spent undertaking basic RN training which includes naval procedures and practice. This period of training is undertaken at HMS Raleigh near Plymouth. Each new arrival is entered into a division. The RN division system offers a support network; every new recruit is given a division officer to whom they can turn with personal problems.

Upon completion of the basic training course at HMS Raleigh, new recruits spend a two-week period on the Medical Branch Acquaint Course at RNH Haslar before commencing duties. Duties could include serving at a shore-based hospital (QARNNs rarely serve at sea during peacetime), or accompanying Marines on exercise in Norway.

RN second level nurses have the opportunity to undertake the conversion course whether trained in the RN or direct entry; each applicant is considered on their own merits. Within the clearly defined ranking system there is ample opportunity for the second level nurse to gain promotion from the grade of Able Rate to Chief Petty Officer. This is a separate career structure to that of the nursing profession. It is interesting to note that of the four ranks between Able Rate and Chief Petty Officer the first level general nurse has to proceed through three of them. There is considerable overlap which enables the committed enrolled nurse who works hard to be promoted on merit within the naval structure.

All successful nursing applicants undertake an Open Engagement with the RN. In practice this means that an individual can serve for up to twenty-two years with the opportunity to give eighteen months' notice after two-and-a-half years' service.

The RN actively encourages the second level nurse to undertake further professional and naval training. The opportunity to move from specialty areas to general areas of nursing is widely available and the RN encourages nurses to keep their broad nursing skills up to date.

Details of opportunities allied to nursing can be obtained from the Director of the Navy Careers Service or the nearest Royal Navy and Royal Marines Careers Office. A list of Navy Careers Information

Offices can be obtained from the publication *Methods of Entry* C.P.3, October 1991.

Director of Nursing Services (RAF),
Room 515, Ministry of Defence, First Avenue House, High Holborn, London WC1 6HE.
Matron in Chief, QARNNS,
First Avenue House, High Holborn, London WC1 6HE.
QARANC Liaison Officer,
Ministry of Defence, Army, DAR 2, Room 1113, Empress State Building, Lillie Road, London SW6 1TR.
The Director,
Naval Careers Service, Old Admiralty Building, Spring Gardens, London SW1A 2BE.

7

Nursing in the Prison Service

Caring for people in prison is one of the most exciting challenges in nursing today. Increasingly the Prison Service sees itself as providing a caring service that rehabilitates offenders. Nurses play a large part in this process.

Many prison officers choose to become nurses within the Prison Service and undertake the relevant training in order to extend their skills. Qualified nurses entering the Prison Service do not have to undertake further nurse training but are required to undertake a ten-week officer training course, a residential course in either Rugby or Wakefield. The course includes such skills as personal safety, controlling inmates and interpreting non-verbal communication.

The work is extremely hard but very rewarding. Much of the caring is psychological; rebuilding confidence, helping prisoners to discuss their problems and worries, helping to turn a negative experience into a positive one and equip them for life outside.

Many prisons are being rebuilt and upgraded and new prisons are currently being built. The Prison Service itself is constantly being upgraded and the most self-disciplined and caring of people are being sought to enhance the service.

Working closely with medical officers, prison officers and other agencies, the hospital officer produces a plan of care for each prisoner that will take account of all the individual's needs.

Nursing in the female prisons brings with it the challenges of running mother and baby units, obstetric and gynaecology work and the chance to help distressed women.

Nursing within male prisons has different challenges but can include care for individuals undergoing surgical, as well as psychiatric, treatment.

There are different types of prisons and care needs. This is evident from the range of activities and skills that are required from applicants. Further details about nursing in the Prison Service can be obtained from the Prison Service Headquarters in London.

Individual posts are advertised in the nursing press as they arise; the service does not recruit for prisons in general.

Second level opportunities

For both second level nurse general and second level nurses with psychiatric training the opportunities are expanding. There is the possibility of moving into a prison officer role from the hospital officer role and continuing up the ladder to Governor status. Conversion to first level nurse is considered on an individual basis. The Prison Service does not provide conversion course training but may be willing to help a nurse with secondment or open learning conversion.

First level nurse opportunities

The first level nurse in the Prison Service may enjoy promotion fairly quickly and could soon find himself/herself in charge of a small unit. Skills that are required include the usual clinical or psychiatric skills and the ability to motivate and lead a team in sometimes difficult circumstances. Promotion is granted upon ability and examinations followed by an interview.

The opportunity to progress into management and administration is one which some officers choose to apply for. Staff support and effective management of resources in the Prison Service are as important as caring for the prisoners. Becoming a senior nurse in the Prison Service gives nurses an opportunity to help select the right kind of staff and to develop a setting for both staff and prisoners that is conducive to effective rehabilitation. There is a strong emphasis upon staff development.

USEFUL ADDRESSES

HM Prison Service Headquarters,
    Cleland House, Page Street, London SW1P 4LN.
Scottish Office Home and Health Department,
    Prison Service Recruitment (Nursing) Room 115D, Calton House, 5
    Redheughs Rigg, Edinburgh EH12 9HW.

8

Charge Nurse/Ward Sister/Manager

THE RESPONSIBILITIES

The role is a demanding and rewarding one which carries ultimate immediate responsibility for the effective use of resources such as stock, equipment and manpower (sometimes exclusively nursing, in other instances including ward maids, ward clerks, department assistants and other people attached to the unit). On occasions the role could also include responsibility for a budget. This may be exercised in the form of direct responsibility, or could involve influence over part or all of the budget. The benefits of budget holding include the opportunity to control expenditure more effectively.

Delegating work to members of the team according to their skills, abilities and qualifications is a key responsibility of the charge nurse/sister. The ability to be able to delegate jobs and responsibilities that could be done better by yourself is sometimes difficult but essential, if other members of the team are to develop new skills and the charge nurse/sister is to find time for the many other things now required from the role. Delegation can be practised by senior staff nurses left in charge of the ward. These occasions should be used as a good opportunity to practise the skill for nurses contemplating a move from the staff nurse grade to sister/charge nurse.

Coordinating patient care by delegating the individual patient's care to named nurses and partly by liaising with other disciplines, management and services is an aspect of the sister/charge nurse's role which is being delegated much more, a situation which some post holders find difficult to handle but not impossible to overcome. Delegation of care should be undertaken mindful of the *Code of Professional Conduct* and *The Scope of Professional Practice* guidelines (UKCC 1992).

Administration takes increasingly more of the time allotted to this role, not only of the day to day business but plans for the future. In an era in which organizations require large amounts of sophisticated information in order to be able to price care and plan services, the charge nurse/sister is inevitably the individual who is able to provide the most information about nursing care in the workplace. Not all the administration concerns the requirements of outside bodies; some of it is straightforward handling of issues such as the duty roster, over-seeing stocks, supplies and handling patients' possessions. Control of environmental conditions such as heating, lighting, noise, cleanliness and ventilation is not directly achieved by the charge nurse/sister but are things that should be regularly monitored in the interests of patients and staff alike.

Leading clinical practice is an essential part of the role. As role model in the immediate area, members of the nursing team look towards the charge nurse/sister for inspiration, support, leadership and an example to follow. While increasingly more time is being taken up with non-clinical activities, the individual within the role usually has the most advanced clinical skills in the immediate area. The implementation of new research-based practice and participation in practice development are part of the job.

Good communications within the ward/area are vital and often mark the difference between happy, coordinated teams and demotivated, uncoordinated teams: Matthews (1987) lists communication breakdown as one of the causes of stress in nursing. Regular ward meetings with individuals and checking that methods and lines of communication are successful are all part of the role. Beyond the immediate team communications with other disciplines, management and professional organizations help to keep the nursing staff both informed and able to respond appropriately. Networking with outside agencies such as special interest groups can have significant benefits.

Morale and staff welfare play a major part in the success of any patient care area. Low morale results in a higher turnover of staff, absenteeism and apathy. High morale tends to engender commitment, enthusiasm, low sickness and low absenteeism. Staff that feel valued and cared for stay longer and deliver better quality care. Patients often comment upon issues such as the nurse's workload and happiness.

Burnout in the nursing profession is a process which can occur as a result of excessive stress; it may occur in the individual nurse or may be present in the entire team. In either case it is the responsibility of the charge nurse/ward sister to identify the causes and give or seek assistance to alleviate problems in the interests of staff team health and wellbeing. Lack of support, patient suffering, constant change and low staffing levels are all causes of burnout within teams and individuals.

Signs and symptoms include resistance to change, absenteeism, anxiety, fatigue and conflict, to name but a few. Nurses considering a career move into the charge nurse/sister role should study stress in nursing and try to identify mechanisms that they could employ to alleviate or avoid these problems within the team.

Staff selection and appointment are undertaken in cooperation with the nurse manager and personnel department. Both the charge nurse/ sister and manager will have ideas about the skills and qualifications required to fill a post, along with the type of personality that will enhance the team and help it to grow.

THE INDIVIDUAL

Charge nurses/sisters are usually selected by nurse managers in cooperation with other bodies, such as the team medical consultants, and are chosen for a variety of reasons.

The individual chosen must be able to exercise leadership not only as a ward/unit manager but also as a role model and person by whom others are happy to be led. Leadership skills required include the ability to provide support and guidance, justice and compassion and above all, vision.

Vision and direction along with the ability to be able to plan the route are important and highly desirable in the charge nurse/sister today.

A sound body of clinical knowledge is a minimum requirement. Nearly all advertisements for these posts now require a further specialist course, such as an appropriate English National Board qualification. Many employers are increasingly attempting to find nurses that have further qualifications in clinical practice and a degree.

The ability to be able to motivate others by various means is essential. Usually motivation is positive and comes in the form of enthusiasm, praise and support for others along with other reward mechanisms such as recognition and promotion. Occasionally the situation may demand that a member of the staff has to be disciplined. This is one of the least favoured aspects of the role, but handled through the usual formal routes in a sensitive and caring way some disciplinary situations can be positive in their outcome for all concerned.

Individuals in this type of role will need to have not only the skills but the commitment to teaching. Patient education and staff education can be used by the charge nurse/sister not just to communicate infor-mation and ideas but to motivate and gain support for ideas if the necessity arises. Qualifications such as ENB 998/997 or City and Guilds 730 are desirable. Presentation of information is not just a formal process but very much an individual approach. Discover the styles that suit you best.

SUPPORT NETWORKS

The sister/charge nurse needs to identify support networks and mentors from whom he/she can learn. Working as part of a team but being ultimately responsible for that team can be quite stressful, and on occasions lonely. Many Health Authorities and organizations have networks and meetings for sisters and charge nurses to exchange ideas and support. Larger organizations may find this more difficult to achieve because of the numbers involved.

Nursing Times runs sisters' conferences which offer a useful opportunity to meet individuals from other organizations and highlight new developments in the profession and in practice.

THE CHANGING EMPHASIS

There is a move away from individual tasks within a set routine towards delegating whole areas of care to suitably qualified and experienced nurses. Systems such as primary nursing facilitate this method of working and the Audit Commission seems to advocate this method of practice.

As a result of this change in care delivery patterns the sister/charge nurse role has changed from one in which the individual retains control over specific tasks into a role which concentrates upon enabling others to plan and carry out tasks more effectively. The sister/charge nurse role therefore has a much larger component of education and administration than before.

The role looks as though it is likely to develop into two distinct directions in the future.

(1) Clinical leader with administrative back-up in other forms.
(2) Administrative manager with clinical expertise.

Although Friend (1992) notes that the role could be undertaken in a number of different ways.

Current job advertisements reflect the emerging different roles. Varying job descriptions and goals for the post holders indicate the different views of individual organizations. It is important to recognize this when applying for sister/charge nurse posts with another organization.

In any scenario the ward leader exercises considerable personal power and is able to influence the thinking of managers, medical staff, ward staff, patients and their families. It is therefore essential that a sister's/charge nurse's knowledge is current and research-based. Skills that may help a sister/charge nurse to influence others (and thereby gain support and hopefully extra resources) include good written and verbal skills together with a degree of assertiveness and self-confidence. These, combined with the ability to think analytically, provide solutions and listen to others, are some of the qualities of the most successful sister/charge nurse.

Quality assurance, audit of nursing, health care assistant training, resource management and many other initiatives have all bitten heavily into the ward leader's time and role. Increasingly, the sister/charge nurse has to manage the changes and develop the staff, ward and care accordingly. A large part of the sister/charge nurse role is likely to be devoted to developing systems, people and practice. Some of this will be as a result of professional and legislative requirements; other elements are likely to be generated by enthused ward staff themselves.

Clearly, recent legislation and professional initiatives such as nursing development units are forcing wards and units to move away from traditional routines and approach a much more fluid and developmental situation led by dynamic individuals. Individuals wishing to become sister/charge nurse need to analyse their own leadership skills and commitment with this in mind.

Undoubtedly the sister/charge nurse is one of the most rewarding roles within nursing. The opportunity to influence and develop care while remaining in the clinical setting is often quoted as one of the more rewarding elements of the job.

Anyone contemplating a move into the sister/charge nurse role should try to have some knowledge of the key people that he/she will be working with. Senior nurses, therapists and consultants all have to be worked with and their support needs to be gained for most of the larger projects that a ward undertakes; knowledge of these individuals may help you to decide whether this is the job for you or not.

The overall effect seems to be that the traditional image of a sister/charge nurse has practically disappeared. The role is undergoing the same changes that happened to the senior nurse roles once the traditional matron disappeared. Evaluation of individual job contents, their value to the organization and the need for change has to be juggled with the benefits of stability, continuity and confidence. Articles by Booth (1992), Scadden (1992) and Sills (1992) all have marginally conflicting views upon budget holding and administration, but all reflect the general trend towards these preoccupations within the role.

REFERENCES

Booth B (1992) Someone to believe in. *Nursing Times*, **88**(15): 36–7.
Friend B (1992) Sisterhood is powerful. *Nursing Times*, **88**(8): 24–9.

Matthews A (1987) *In Charge of the Ward.* Oxford: Blackwell.
Scadden G (1992) Ward budgeting. *Nursing Times,* **88**(11): 35–8.
Sills E (1992) Keeping a high profile. *Nursing Times,* **88**(25): 36–7.
UKCC (1992) *Code of Professional Conduct.* London: UKCC.
UKCC (1992) *The Scope of Professional Practice.* London: UKCC.

USEFUL READING

Allen H (1982) *The Ward Sister: Role and Preparation.* London: Baillière Tindall.
Armstrong M (1981) *Practical Nurse Management.* London: Edward Arnold.
Audit Commission (1992) *Making Time for Patients: a Handbook for Ward Sisters.* London: Audit Commission.
Bailey R D (1985) *Coping with Stress in Caring.* Oxford: Blackwell.
Bond M (1986) *Stress and Self Awareness: a Guide for Nurses.* London: Heinemann.
Burnard P (1991) *Coping with Stress in the Health Professions: a Practical Guide.* London: Chapman and Hall.
Hinchcliffe S M (ed) (1986) *Teaching Clinical Nursing.* Edinburgh: Churchill Livingstone.
Lemin B (1977) *First Line Management.* Tunbridge Wells: Pitman.
Matthews A (1987) *In Charge of the Ward.* Oxford: Blackwell.
McConnell E (1982) *Burnout in the Nursing Profession: Coping Strategies, Causes and Costs.* London: Mosby.
Pembry S (1980) *The Ward Sister: Key to Nursing.* London: Royal College of Nursing.
Perry E (ed) (1978) *Ward Management and Teaching,* 2nd edn. London: Baillière Tindall.
Runciman P (1983) *Ward Sister at Work.* Edinburgh: Churchill Livingstone.
Stewart N (1992) For better or worse. *Nursing Times,* **88**(20): 36–7.
Vaughan B & Pillmoor M (eds) (1989) *Managing Nursing Work.* London: Scutari Press.
Waits J (1985) *Budgetary Control: a Guide for Nurse Managers.* London: Health Services Manpower Review.
Young A (1990) *The Law and Professional Conduct in Nursing.* London: Scutari Press.

USEFUL ADDRESS

National Ward Sisters Conference Organizers,
    MacMillan Conferences, 4 Little Essex Street, London WC2R 3LF.

9

Senior Nurse Opportunities

Beyond ward-based nursing, senior nurse roles vary from establishment to establishment. Organizations have different visions of the role of senior nurses and their particular position within the hierarchy. Nurse managers have a recognizable place in the hierarchy of most organizations and most administrators, nurses and medics have some understanding of the nurse manager's role. Other senior nurse roles such as clinical nurse specialist, project nurse and staff development officers have a less easily identifiable place in systems and are sometimes not 'recognized' by others in the system, although this is rapidly changing in the light of the major contribution that these roles are making to innovative practice.

In general, the future of the senior nurse role lies in the ability to move away from traditional methods of working towards innovative and democratic methods. The maintenance manager who concentrates energy upon 'day to day' decisions and personnel issues is being gradually replaced by managers whose roles are to develop the service, systems and staff in a much more dynamic and strategic way. Everyday management is being increasingly devolved to the ward manager/sister level. Other senior nurse roles such as clinical nurse specialists, whose roles do not include management issues, are free to develop strategy, systems and service much more rapidly.

The content of individual senior nurse roles are a direct reflection of the organization's vision, both of nursing within the system and the contribution that nursing will be making to the organization's vision for care and goals to that purpose. Central to the success of each senior nurse's role are the issues that surround leadership skills and scope. Both the ability and opportunity to fashion and execute the role are determined by the qualities of the individual in the role and constraints placed upon them.

Senior nurse roles have a very significant number of medium- and long-term goals (some taking months or years) that only inch forward on a daily basis, and are often projects that others standing in temporarily for the senior nurse therefore do not become fully involved with. This major element of medium- and long-term work in the senior nurse's role represents a significant departure from the immediate clinical setting roles, such as ward sister, where the goals are much more short-term and results highly visible on a daily basis. This aspect of a senior nurse's role can be frustrating and disappointing to the nurse moving into a senior nurse position, unaware of the need to change their thinking about achievement within the job.

Mindful of the above, individuals seeking to move into a senior nurse role should look beyond the title and job description into the organization itself in great depth before making the move. Many organizations produce job descriptions that are a checklist of responsibilities and tasks, when in actual fact they require the role to meet certain goals in the future. In some instances, individuals are free to develop the role in the manner that they choose as long as goals are met. Individuals who do not perceive this aspect of the role may feel unsupported. Equally, individuals who accept a post that has activities solely confined to the responsibilities and tasks identified in the job description, which are managed in a specified way, may be frustrated. It is therefore important to establish a shared vision of the role beyond the job description and to be sure that your leadership style is compatible with the organization's vision for the role.

Essential reading for anybody contemplating a move into a senior nurse role is the Audit Commission's (1991) examination of various senior nurse roles in the report *The Virtue of Patients*. This sensitive survey of the way various organizations within the health service have interpreted and used senior nurse roles, along with trends for the future of the role, is invaluable.

A good understanding of the UKCC *Code of Professional Conduct, Exercising Accountability* and *The Scope of Professional Practice* (UKCC 1992) coupled with the ability to apply them to practice are essential.

Senior nurse roles offer some of the most rewarding opportunities currently available in nursing. The chance to develop practice, enhance patient care and motivate a cared-for team of nurses is not to be underestimated. This type of leadership opportunity can come through either direct line management or other senior nurse roles.

Opportunities beyond the senior nurse middle management bracket discussed here include general management, directors of nursing service and chief nursing officer roles at senior management levels within the organization.

Qualifications for senior nurse roles vary according to the exact nature of the role and organization. Increasingly, most senior nurses have degrees and are working for higher degrees. Senior nurses employed within certain roles, such as clinical nurse specialist and professional development, require additional qualifications that are relevant, such as specialist English National Board courses and education qualifications.

Broad management qualifications can be useful for all these roles and two particularly good courses that are both relevant and dynamic in their content are the Open University's 'Managing Voluntary and Non-profit Making Enterprises' (part of the certificate course) and the course entitled 'Winning Resources and Support', ideal for those who are interested in finding money for their unit and professional activities. The National Health Service Training Directorate run a number of management training schemes. Workshops, full courses and open learning initiatives are just some of the methods of delivery. A number of these courses are run in conjunction with other agencies such as the Open University. Some courses have bursaries attached to them. Further details can be obtained from the Training Directorate.

NURSE MANAGEMENT

A nurse manager is an advanced practitioner who exercises leadership and some degree of control over a team of nurses. The roles are interpreted differently according to the organization but usually include some of the following elements: staffing issues such as employment interviews and shortlisting; dismissal; individual performance review; budgeting, either direct control of the budget, the power to delegate it, or influence over part of it. Project developments and the management of change are key issues; building and maintaining integrated teams of nurses; providing vision and direction for the team along with leadership and motivation; negotiation and bridging between higher and lower levels of nurses, medical and nursing staff, nursing and administration; counselling individuals and supporting teams; creating the right culture to enable the team and individuals along with nursing practice to grow.

Quality assurance issues include audit. The nurse manager is accountable for the total nursing service within the designated unit. In addition to maintaining and improving standards of patient care the nurse manager has a duty to have due regard for the workload of nurses. An interest in the skill mix and staffing levels in relationship to the required patient care is often part of the nurse manager's role. Nurse information systems and supplying much more complex and detailed information about nursing activity may fall within the remit of a nurse manager.

Increasingly, the role of the nurse manager is moving towards a more strategic approach, some of the tasks mentioned above being delegated elsewhere. The future of the unit, developing staff and care delivery take increasingly more time, along with the need to facilitate and manage many of the changes that are directed at nursing from outside of the unit.

Personal qualities that match the job are important in these roles. The ability to be able to enthuse and motivate people to change, together with the organizational skills required to manage yourself, your time and others are essential.

CLINICAL NURSE SPECIALIST

An advanced practitioner with a high level of expertise, the clinical nurse specialist is a leader in a very different way to the nurse manager. Reliant upon the ability of the individual in the job to lead by example and motivation, the role moves other nurses forward with it. Using sound research-based knowledge, often applied to a patient caseload, the clinical nurse specialist is a mentor and role model.

The clinical nurse specialist has a commitment to staff and patient education, often teaching and acting as a resource for all. Networking with other individuals in similar roles is important, as is sharing information and support with each other. The clinical nurse specialist often works independently and is usually the only senior nurse in the organization to have that particular role.

The role has been interpreted in different ways in different organizations and is of varying worth to each place. This is reflected in the grading, degree of autonomy and responsibilities that the individual is given. These roles cross boundaries whatever the grade of the individual in post. Clinical nurse specialists may be advising chief nurses and addressing conferences one day, teaching a health care assistant the next.

The success of these roles is dependent upon the characteristics of the individual and their ability to develop the specialty as a whole. Assertive, well presented, highly organized enthusiasts who are good communicators and can work well on their own are most likely to succeed.

Not uncommonly, nurses in these types of roles express feelings of uncertainty about their performance and feel unsupported. Being clear about the exact job content can be a problem for clinical nurse specialists. There is a need for individual clinical nurse specialists to have a clearly defined role even if they have to define it themselves beyond the job description. Lines of accountability should be clear and a shared vision is important. These issues are not a disincentive, merely a feature of unique roles with dynamic individuals within them, and indicate the role's dependence upon clear goals and personal qualities as opposed to a manifestation of tasks and responsibilities.

NURSE ADVISERS

The nurse adviser comes in many guises and is another role that is often unique to the individual organization in the exact job content. Some have a major clinical input, others are much more traditionally management-based. Each job has to be considered by the applicant as a unique role.

An advanced practitioner with highly developed leadership skills, the nurse adviser works across boundaries of grade and discipline. The role has less of the mentor and role model element found in the clinical nurse specialist and more of a preceptor, enabler and facilitator role. There is a strong commitment to education and perhaps staff development. The nurse adviser is less of a specialist and more of a generalist, able to turn their hand to many aspects of enabling, change management and strategic advancements. In common with some other senior nurse roles, the adviser's role may overlap with others and is usually a non-line management job. The grades and remits of the adviser's role reflect the organization's vision of the role and overall objectives. In common with other roles, there are the usual frustrations and enjoyments of being in a relatively independent and unique situation. There is a need to be clear about the nature and content of these roles and to have clear objectives.

On occasions, this type of role may be coupled with management responsibilities. Such roles are often line management posts with a strong clinical/advisory element.

PROJECT NURSE/SUPPORT NURSE

These are senior nurse posts that have boundaries that may overlap with other roles, and the job content varies considerably. An advanced practitioner who is usually attached to a line manager, the project and support nurse usually has much more clearly defined job content than clinical nurse specialists and advisers. These roles may be a direct continuation of line managers' goals and roles and can enjoy less autonomy than the specialists and advisers, who operate outside line management, sometimes with differing goals. A strong part of the project and support nurse's role is to translate ideas into action of whatever kind and act as a bridge between people on occasion. Sometimes senior nurses are employed in these roles for general duties and sometimes for specific jobs. These roles are usually an excellent stepping stone into line management and may involve acting for the line managers in their absence.

The exact role depends upon the size and nature of the organization. Individuals are employed for a number of reasons, sometimes for a sole specific purpose, such as officer for cardio-pulmonary resuscitation training. Sometimes the role may be part of a team developing a range of staff in a variety of subjects and ways. Sole practitioners may be employed to coordinate the service and programmes and to identify needs. On occasion the role may be a key organizational post with wide-ranging powers such as the BUPA Professional Development Officer.

There is a strong commitment to both the service and education needs as well as individual development. Career development advice seems to be part of this job and the individual usually has an informal counselling role for the staff. The Post Registration Education and Practice proposal (UKCC 1990) is likely to increase the need for this type of senior nurse.

Skills required include the ability to be well organized, self-motivating, a good communicator and to have excellent presentation skills. The staff development officer/inservice training officer is an advanced practitioner.

LECTURER/PRACTITIONER

Some organizations have developed a role that is primarily clinical and workplace based. As part of the clinical team the lecturer/practitioner has a specific clinical input coupled with a formal commitment to staff development. Lecturing outside the clinical area may also be a feature of this type of role.

For the nurse who enjoys teaching and staff development but wishes to retain a firm clinical commitment, this type of role could be extremely rewarding.

CONSULTANT NURSE

Practised by a few who are pioneers and leaders, the consultant nurse is becoming more evident in nursing. Acting as a catalyst for particular aspects of nursing, the individuals occupy roles that are virtually created by themselves. Pushing aside traditional thinking, the consultant nurse advances nursing by various means, many of which are unconventional, and as a result is generally respected and acknowledged well beyond the immediate job. The consultant nurse is probably somebody for whom a job description could not be written, the individual and role being far too dynamic. Observation of some practising consultant nurses suggests that there is a strong missionary element about the consultant nurse role which includes 'spreading the word' by various means. Conferences, seminars, publishing books and writing articles are often involved. The immensity of the task of 'spreading the word' nationally through a 600,000-plus workforce of nurses requires a business-like approach to their work. These individuals are leaders within the profession and unlike all of the other roles discussed in this volume, this is a role which cannot possibly be applied for and probably can only be created by the individual themselves, whatever their status. The consultant nurse creates a 'niche' for themselves for the duration of their mission.

REFERENCE

Audit Commission (1991) *The Virtue of Patients: Making Best Use of Ward Nursing Resources.* London: HMSO.

USEFUL READING

Armitage P & Burnard P (1991) Mentors or preceptors? Narrowing the theory/practice gap. *Nurse Education Today,* **11**: 225–9.
Bowman M (1986) *Nurse Management and Education: a Conceptual Approach to Change.* London: Croom Helm.
Castledine G (1991a) The advanced nurse practitioner part one. *Nursing Standard,* **5**(43): 34–6.
Castledine G (1991b) The advanced nurse practitioner part two. *Nursing Standard,* **5**(44): 33–5.
Davidson L & Cole A (1991) A crisis of leadership. *Nursing Times,* **87**(1): 22–5.
Douglas L & Bevis E (1983) *Nursing Management and Leadership in Action,* 4th edn. London: Mosby.
Hameric A & Spross J (eds) (1989) *The Clinical Nurse Specialist in Theory and Practice,* 2nd edn. London: Saunders.
Marriner A (ed) (1982) *Contemporary Nursing Management: Issues and Practice.* London: Mosby.
Rowden R (1984) *Managing Nursing.* London: Baillière Tindall.
Strafford R (1991) The evolution of the specialist. *Nursing Times,* **87**(16): 38–40.
Stewart A & Stewart V (1981) *Tomorrow's Managers Today.* London: IPM.
UKCC (1992) *Code of Professional Conduct.* London: UKCC.

UKCC (1992) *Exercising Accountability*. London: UKCC.
UKCC (1992) *The Scope of Professional Practice*. London: UKCC.
UKCC (1990) *The Report of the Post-Registration Education and Practice Project*. London: UKCC.

USEFUL JOURNAL

Senior Nurse, Nursing Standard Publications, Harrow.

USEFUL ADDRESSES

National Health Service Training Directorate,
  St Bartholomew's Court, 18 Christmas Street, Bristol BS1 5BT.
Open University
  Walton Hall, Milton Keynes MK7 6AA.

10

Opportunities for Nurses with a Degree

Research posts occur at all levels and in many disciplines. The posts may involve teamwork investigating particular conditions, the nurse being required to collect raw data in various forms. Other posts may be entirely independent, the employed nurse undertaking the complete project from start to finish, answerable only to a steering committee. The more junior posts tend to be part of a team effort. Senior research posts, attracting higher salaries, usually require much more experience and extensive research skills to develop a project independently.

Nurses contemplating research as a career need to analyse the route through which they might progress and to select a suitable starting post accordingly. Participation in medical research can be a useful experience but it may prove difficult to progress beyond a certain level. Nursing research now has a rapidly developing career structure, from small projects undertaken on secondment from the ward area to opportunities in the Department of Health or in a university.

Private companies that recruit clinical trials research nurses offer an opportunity to gain insight within research, but the career development potential for this type of employment is not clear.

Occasionally, nurses can persuade managers to release them from clinical duties for a short period to undertake research into such subjects as nursing care outcomes, patient expectations of service and experiences. Projects such as these contribute to the quality of patient care and may be particularly useful at a time when new services are being planned. The clinical nurse who has graduate status and skills is well placed to undertake such projects.

Projects that are generated within an organization by the organization itself are usually offered to internal candidates. Nurses who generate such a project may be given secondment or a time allowance to undertake the piece of work.

Advertisements for nurses required to participate in medical research projects or undertake a major piece of work are usually advertised in the nursing press.

EMPLOYMENT WITHIN DIFFERENT DISCIPLINES

The nurse graduate is able to transfer his or her skills into other disciplines with relative ease. Nurse tutors and health educationalists are examples of occupations allied to nursing for which graduate nursing status is useful and in the case of nurse tutor, obligatory.

Graduate status may help entry into other professions such as physiotherapy, occupational therapy and medicine. The nursing degree will probably enable the nurse to undertake a shortened course in some instances, but this needs to be negotiated on an individual basis with the training institution.

Some of the analytical skills required in management are gained during undergraduate education and could be transferred into general management. The National Health Service Training Directorate provide a graduate entry fast-track training for would-be Health Service managers. Successful graduate entrants who complete the training can be in positions of considerable responsibility within a relatively short period of time. Further details of this can be acquired from the National Health Service Training Unit.

SELF-GENERATED OPPORTUNITIES

Many graduates of nursing may choose to develop their clinical experience and career but use their graduate skills to enhance the role. Small studies carried out in the workplace could lead to improvements in care; publishing the results and experiences can be both rewarding and have an element of financial gain.

Writing for publications is not confined to nurse graduates, but undoubtedly the skills gained while undertaking undergraduate research help an individual to produce a polished piece of written work and a valued piece of research. Most journals require a constant supply of ethically sound, clinical, educational and management material. Interesting and informative articles help to attract readership. Current topics are most likely to be published, as are innovatory and mildly controversial issues. The major journals regularly publish guide-lines for contributors which detail the length and style of a submission. Further details and guidance can be obtained from the journals' editors.

Careful examination of published articles including content, layout and references can help the would-be author.

Successful writers of short articles are often approached by journals for further work and in some instances manage to earn a small regular income. The length of time between an article being submitted to a journal until its publication can be quite considerable. Writers should not be dismayed by this but continue to develop their new skills by writing more articles after the first one has been accepted. Rejection of an article can be for a number of reasons, including poor writing style, inaccurate content or of low interest to the journal's client group. Most journals now give some type of feedback to the author so that they can act accordingly.

Writing a book for publication is a major undertaking. Most authors submit a proposal detailing intended length, content, purpose of the volume and proposed readership to the publisher before work begins. The proposal and a couple of chapters are then sent out for review to acknowledged experts. Depending upon the thoughts of the experts, the probable market interest and other considerations, the commissioning editor will reject or accept the proposal. If the proposal is accepted a contract is drawn up and work proceeds. Mindful of the large resources in terms of time, material for content and maybe even payment for secretarial work the would-be author needs to be sure that they can make the commitment.

HIGHER DEGREES AND FURTHER STUDIES

The nurse graduate, by virtue of graduate status, is able to proceed to undertaking higher degrees by further study or research. Undertaking Masters degrees and Doctorates can be coupled with employers' goals for care if the further degree is undertaken on a part-time basis. Research based in the workplace, and taken with recommendations back into workplace practice, can be a means of justifying expenditure on higher degrees and improving care at the same time.

Some nurse graduates may wish to transfer their first degree into a different type of postgraduate study such as the various Health Service postgraduate diplomas that are available in various universities.

The Post Registration Education and Practice scheme envisages that in future all nurses will work through graduate status to postgraduate status and beyond as their career develops.

ACADEMIC EMPLOYMENT

For some nurse graduates the desired way forward may be into academic employment. Most universities now have health studies departments and many have nursing sections. Employment in the academic world can be found in a number of ways. Lecturers are usually postgraduate appointments and continued research is seen as part of the role. Some universities offer paid post-doctoral research posts. These are usually fixed-term appointments within an amount of funding that has been raised for a particular piece of work. Some individuals undertaking post-doctoral and postgraduate research can attract further income by giving occasional lectures to undergraduates. Lectureships have a slightly greater security of tenure, although this is rapidly changing. The career structure is then through the education system and into higher education management posts, such as Vice Principal and Dean of the faculty.

ENTRY INTO OTHER PROFESSIONS

Graduate status in nursing can be used to gain entry into training for other professions on a short course. Teacher training for the graduate is considerably shortened in the form of the Postgraduate Certificate of Education (PGCE). Further details of this can be obtained from the Department of Education.

Entry into the legal profession for graduates is considerably shortened. The academic stage of a lawyer's training is reduced from a three-year full-time (five-year part-time) course in law to a one-year full-time (two-year part-time) course for a graduate with a non-law degree. The practical training for lawyers remains the same for those that have done the full three years in law and those who have taken the common professional examination. Further details of these courses and others are available from universities and local libraries.

USEFUL READING

Albert T (1990) *Medical Journalism: The Writer's Guide.* Oxford: Radcliffe Press.

Cormack D (1984) *Writing for Nursing and Allied Professions.* London: Blackwell.

Findon M (1992) *Roget Register of Graduate Employment and Training.* Manchester: Central Services Unit.

USEFUL JOURNALS

Health Services Journal, Macmillan Magazines, London.
Nursing Standard, Scutari Projects, Harrow.
Nursing Times, Macmillan Magazines, London.
Times Educational Supplement, News International plc, London.

General

Association of Graduate Recruiters,
  Sheraton House, Castle Park, Cambridge CB3 0AX.
Central Services Unit (publications for graduates),
  Armstrong House, Oxford Road, Manchester M1 7ED.
Kogan Page (Career Publications),
  120 Pentonville Road, London N1 9JN.

Research

Nursing Research Index,
  Room 5E05, Department of Health, Quarry House, Quarry Hill, Leeds LS2 7UD.
Research Special Interest Group,
  c/o The Royal College of Nursing, 20 Cavendish Square, London W1M 0AB.

Law

The Bar Council,
  11 South Square, Gray's Inn, London WC1R 5EL.
The Civil Service Commission,
  Alençon Link, Basingstoke, Hampshire RG21 1JB.
The Law Society,
  The Law Society Hall, 113 Chancery Road, London WC2A 1PL.
The Council of Legal Education,
  39 Eagle Street, London WC1R 4AJ.

MAJOR GRADUATE EMPLOYERS

Audit Commission,
  Nicholson House, Lime Kiln Close, Stoke Gifford, Bristol BS12 6SU.
British Airways,
  Meadow Bank, PO Box 59, Hounslow, Middlesex TW5 9QX.
BBC Corporate Recruitment,
  Broadcasting House, London W1A 1AA.
Butlins Ltd,
  Bognor Regis, West Sussex PO21 1JJ.
Chartfield Enterprises (Medical Recruitment),
  Parkside House, 17 East Parade, Harrogate, Yorkshire HG1 5LF.
Coopers and Lybrand Deloitte,
  Plumtree Court, London EC4A 4HT.

Ethical Register,
 Innovex House, Reading Road, Henley-on-Thames, Oxfordshire RG9
 1EL.
Halifax Building Society,
 Trinity Road, Halifax, West Yorkshire HX1 2RG.
ICI plc,
 Group Recruitment, PO Box 90, Wilton, Middlesbrough, Cleveland
 TS5 8JE.
Marks and Spencer plc,
 Michael House, 47–57 Baker Street, London W1A 1DN.
Graduate Recruitment,
 Pfizer Central Research, Pfizer, Sandwich, Kent CT13 9NJ.
Police Service,
 Home Office, Queen Anne's Gate, London SW1H 9AT.
Smith and Nephew plc,
 PO Box 81, Hessle Road, Hull, Humberside HU3 2BN.
Wellcome Foundation,
 Temple Hill, Dartford, Kent DA1 5AH.

11

Opportunities Abroad

Overseas opportunities for qualified nurses are numerous, both in quantity and variety, although the range available to second level nurses is not as great as those for first level nurses. Employment can be found as a volunteer, on travel exchange schemes, through employment agencies or as a direct contract with companies that provide health care services abroad.

A regular, useful publication that has occasional opportunities for nurses to work abroad in either seasonal or permanent positions is *Overseas Jobs Express* published fortnightly: for subscription details write directly to them. Vacation Work publish a considerable range of books and directories for people who wish to work abroad in a number of capacities. Two particularly useful volumes, *The Directory of Jobs and Careers Abroad* and *Summer Jobs Abroad*, both contain details of travel, visas, types of work and other information about working and living abroad. A number of the jobs advertised will be suitable for nurses who are willing to work in capacities that utilize their skills but may not necessarily be direct nursing, such as *au pair* work.

For nurses who would like a complete change of direction there are numerous opportunities, from hotel and catering in Germany to agricultural work in Australia, where the wages are high and the cost of living comparatively low. Taking a different temporary job abroad is a good way to find out about the country itself and permanent jobs if you wish to stay.

Working abroad is a tremendous challenge and requires personal courage. Plan the trip carefully, be absolutely clear about the type of work that you are about to undertake and the terms and conditions of employment. Make sure that you have the right amount and type of health care insurance for your destination. Full details and forms can be obtained from your local Department of Health and Social Security or the Benefits Agency, overseas branch. Employment offices and Job Centres have copies of the pamphlet *Working Abroad* which has, among other things, details of work permits and taxation.

The Organization for Economic Cooperation and Development (OECD) has an international clearing house for vacancies, and operates in Britain through your local Job Centre. Job Centres also have details of vacancies advertised by other European Community member states. The Professional and Executive Register publish a weekly magazine (*Executive Post*) which gives details of some international vacancies for professionals. More information about this can be obtained from your nearest Job Centre or the Overseas Placing Unit, Sheffield. Other bodies that may be of help include the Crown Agents for Overseas Governments and Administration, who liaise with over 100 governments and 200 public authorities placing suitably qualified professionals.

VOLUNTARY WORK

Voluntary work is available mainly in the developing countries or countries that are in a state of emergency. It is important to be clear about the reasons for your interest in voluntary work and the particular skills and experience that you have to offer. An understanding of your own strengths and weaknesses is vital if you are to undertake work as a volunteer. Voluntary work is an occupation which demands total commitment whatever the frustrations of the situation.

Nurses that have primary health care experience are likely to be particularly useful in developing countries where long-term, large-scale immunization programmes and health education are part of the strategy for health care. Experienced specialists such as HIV health care workers have much to offer to certain parts of Africa and the developing world.

Ophthalmic nurses, midwives, health visitors and paediatric nurses are urgently required both to deliver health care and to train others.

Details of the types of vacancies and the countries in which they can be found, together with some useful information for potential volunteers, can be obtained from Returned Volunteer Action (RVA) who publish a number of useful leaflets. Most of the jobs are created as a result of the Overseas Development Administration (ODA) aid programmes, policies and commitments to the developing world. Current vacancies and further details of individual opportunities can be obtained from the following four specialist agencies.

Catholic Institute for International Relations (CIIR).
International Voluntary Service (IVS).
United Nations Association International Service (UNAIS).
Voluntary Services Overseas (VSO).

Of the four agencies VSO is the largest and most widely advertised.

Volunteers are employed overseas in emergency situations to deal with specific situations, such as natural disasters or the victims of civil wars. Volunteer work of this nature is by definition unpredictable and therefore probably not suitable for individuals looking for security or regular employment. Agencies such as the International Red Cross employ medical and nursing staff who can be called upon at short notice to work in difficult and sometimes life-threatening situations. The skills needed for this type of work are different from those required for long-term work in developing countries. Acute experience such as accident and emergency work, along with critical care and theatre skills, are the most useful. Personal qualities such as good self-control and the ability to work well under pressure are essential.

Oxfam and Save the Children have emergency lists of professionals able to help at short notice with famine disasters and widespread disease. The East European Partnership, a VSO initiative, is currently seeking nurses to give care and to train local workers. There is a small salary attached to this employment but in essence it remains voluntary work.

TRAVEL EXCHANGE SCHEMES AND SCHOLARSHIPS

Exchange schemes within Europe and the Commonwealth are becoming much more popular as national boundaries become easier to cross and the desire to look at systems and practise elsewhere is growing. Exchanges can be, and are, arranged for groups or individuals. A small number of enterprising organizations in the United Kingdom have arranged exchange visits to other countries for the purpose of study, information or to develop a certain aspect of care. In some instances the cost of the visit is met by the delegates. In other exchanges the organizers have raised funds from various sources to sponsor the exchange.

Exchanges that have been arranged by organizations usually have to be applied for. Would-be applicants need to consider why they want to undertake the experience, what they hope to gain from it and how it will contribute to care. In some cases the organizers will have additional criteria for applicants, particularly if the exchange is funded from charities, and there are criteria for applications attached to the funding.

If the exchange is open to any nurse in the United Kingdom, advertisements appear in the national nursing press. Locally organized exchanges which may have funding attached are usually advertised internally.

Exchange visits can be arranged on an individual basis, although this tends to be a little more difficult and is usually confined to those who go with a specific remit to look at particular aspects of care provision with a view to implementing it here.

It is possible to organize exchange visits for yourself or a group of people if the facility does not exist locally. Be clear about the type of visit you wish to undertake and the reason for it, where you wish to travel and for how long. Contact the Royal College of Nursing International Division for specific advice relating to the country of your choice. Use the international telephone directories for addresses of establishments. Contact the professional organization in the country of your choice for further advice. Make a study of the country and its current health provision. Knowledge of the culture and language would be extremely helpful if not essential in some cases.

Funding or partial funding may be available to help with a project such as this. The funding could be attracted from your employer or organization. It may be applied for from the many charities that sponsor such ventures. Competition for funding from charities is highly competitive.

The Commonwealth Youth Exchange Council funds exchange visits for groups between the ages of sixteen and twenty-five, particularly for the purpose of innovative practice and practice development. Further details can be obtained from the Council.

A variety of charities offer funding to individuals. The Commonwealth Foundation offers funding for professional or skilled persons. The Florence and Don McGregor Trust award finance for travel to enable individuals under thirty-five to have the opportunity to make a contribution to international understanding. The London and Provincial Nursing Services Awards also finance travel abroad; there are few specific criteria for this award, each application being considered on its own merits.

Planning and organizing an exchange visit can be an enjoyable experience, but it requires a great deal of patience and forward thinking. The Royal College of Nursing International Department has a study tour planning service which may be more cost effective for you to use.

Scholarships are frequently advertised in the nursing press for funding that is available nationally. Some scholarships are awarded locally and have specific criteria attached to them. Your local college of nursing library may have details of the smaller local grants available. Scholarships are awarded to individuals who wish to travel abroad for the purpose of study to improve practice and advance knowledge. Scholarships must be applied for and usually have certain criteria; be sure that they apply to you before you apply. It is usual to present a curriculum vitae and aims of the study tour. Some awarding bodies will also want details of how you intend to use the study tour information afterwards and a short report about your visit may be expected. Help with all this may be available from a nurse tutor or manager.

Whether the visit is a scholarship project or exchange it is helpful to keep a diary of events in addition to the other work required. A substantial amount of learning takes place which is not about nursing: different cultures always make an impression! The nurse abroad on a visit or exchange is both a guest and an ambassador about whom people will be curious and keen to learn from, as well as to teach. Try to keep all of the information that you collect clear and well organized. This will help you upon your return when it has to be presented to others.

EMPLOYMENT AGENCIES

Nursing agencies offer some of the best opportunities available abroad. Contracts range from a few days to a number of years in length. The best nursing agencies have a wide variety of vacancies across the world and maintain constant contact with major employers. First level nurses with specialist experience have a good chance of finding a well-paid post in the country of their choice. Dialysis, paediatric skills, intensive care and special care baby unit nurses are among those most commonly requested. Other registered nurses may find that employment is not quite so easy to find, but most nurses with skills that range from psychiatric to medical nursing who have more than a year's experience should be able to find a posting.

Most of the paid employment that nurses are likely to find abroad is in Europe, America, Australia and the Middle East. Contracts in the developing countries such as Africa and India are rare; employment in these areas is usually on a voluntary basis.

Salaries vary according to the value of nursing in each country and the particular post applied for, the status and the skills required. In most of the European countries and America the salaries represent a good living wage and in some countries where nursing has a higher standing than usual (such as Canada), the salary is excellent.

Some of the agencies that specialize in international work or who have departments devoted to it are able to offer nurses some extremely attractive employment packages, which include accommodation of a high standard, induction programmes before and at the beginning of employment, free flights out, back and half-way through the contract. Other packages can include the opportunity to travel from one part of the country to another, changing jobs while abroad. Some of the larger agencies are linked with professional organizations in the country of destination and can provide support for the nurse through this organization locally.

All the reputable agencies will help with insurance cover (some provide it free on certain contracts) for personal accident, medical negligence, indemnity policies and liability. Assistance with obtaining the necessary

travel documents such as visas and passports along with further information about the country of destination is usually part of the agency's
service. Given the potential problems that can arise when working
abroad it is advisable to use one of the reputable nursing agencies who
have extensive experience in international work or a specialist agency.

Employment in the Middle East is available to first level nurses with
a minimum of two years' post-registration experience. Most of the
vacancies are for registered general nurses with specialist experience.
Contracts are usually from three months to one year and can be renewed.
Tax-free salaries, free accommodation and excellent on-site facilities are
just some of the advantages. Personal communication with colleagues
who have worked in the Middle East suggests that many people are
able to enjoy a good lifestyle, and still save considerable sums of money.
The Middle East is rich in culture and tradition, much of which is acces-
sible to the visiting nurse. Local, traditional and religious conventions
are expected to be adhered to by nurses employed within the area.

New Zealand and Australia now advertise fewer vacancies than in
the past, but opportunities still exist. Some individuals may be able
to find employment by contacting hospitals or potential employers
directly. Most will gain employment through an agency. Recently,
both Australia and New Zealand have become much more stringent
about issuing work permits. For the successful nurse, employment in
both New Zealand and Australia offers the opportunity to explore some
wonderful countryside and enjoy a relatively high standard of living.

Switzerland and Holland have opportunities for first level general
nurses with at least one year's post-basic experience. In both cases a
working knowledge of the national language is essential. French or
Dutch to 'O' level/GCSE standard is usually required. Some agencies
offer link language courses for the nurse who is not completely confident about his or her skills.

The United States of America offers some of the most interesting
contracts, with a great deal of variety. Nurses wishing to work in the
United States are expected to have the Commission for Graduate of
Foreign Nursing Schools Certificate (CGFNS) and to have passed the
United States' Board examinations. Some of the major agencies assist
nurses to fly to the United States to take the examinations, help with
education prior to the exams and attend to all necessary paperwork,
which includes obtaining visas and work permits. Nurses may find it
particularly useful to work in the United States and examine health
care systems and delivery in the light of current changes in the British
health care systems.

Private patients require escorts, personal care and support all over
the world. Nursing agencies have contracts for nurses which are tail-
ored to the patient's needs. Each contract is individual and can result

in employment in Italy, France, Belgium, Hong Kong and many other countries that do not usually have opportunities for British nurses. Unlike other forms of employment, this type of work usually requires the nurse to spend a considerable amount of time with one individual; it is therefore worthwhile examining the details of the contract carefully before you go. Amounts of time on duty and off duty should be clear, as should be cover arrangements for off duty periods. The rewards are tremendous and the satisfaction of delivering personal care to a high standard while having the opportunity to travel cannot be underestimated.

The Federation of Recruitment and Employment Services and the Centre for Professional Employment Counselling both have extensive lists detailing hundreds of agencies that have overseas opportunities for nurses. Contact these services directly for further details.

COMPANIES

Some major companies that own and staff health care establishments abroad offer opportunities directly to nurses through the nursing press. The International Hospitals Group have opportunities in the Middle East and America, as do Allied Medical and HCA International. Vacancies are regularly advertised in the nursing journals. A direct approach to the company itself may provide details of the full range of current vacancies.

USEFUL READING

Griffiths S & Legg S (1990) *Au Pair and Nanny's Guide to Working Abroad.* Oxford: Vacation Work.
Jordan's Directories. Jordan's Information Services, Bristol.
Kelly's Business Directories. Kelly's Directories, East Grinstead.
Lipinski A (ed) (1989) *The Directory of Jobs and Careers Abroad.* Oxford: Vacation Work.
Mason P (1992) Smart moves in Zagreb. *Nursing Times,* **33**: 15–17.
Overseas Jobs Express, Brighton.
Woodworth D (ed) (1993) *Summer Jobs Abroad 1993.* Oxford: Vacation Work.

USEFUL ADDRESSES

Action Health,
International Voluntary Health Association,
35 Bird Farm Road, Fulbourn, Cambridge CB1 5DP.

Allied Medical,
  12–18 Grosvenor Gardens, London SW1W 0DZ.
Benefits Agency – Overseas Branch,
  DSS Longbenton, Benton Park Road, Newcastle upon Tyne NE98 1YX.
BNA International,
  443 Oxford Street, London W1N 0NQ.
Catholic Institute for International Relations,
  22 Coleman Fields, London N1 7AF.
Central Bureau for Educational Visits and Exchanges,
  Seymour Mews House, London W1H 9PE.
Centre for Professional Employment Counselling,
  Sundridge Park Management Centre, Plaistow Lane, Bromley, Kent BR1 3JW.
Club Med Recruitment,
  106/110 Brompton Road, London SW3 1JJ.
Crown Agents for Overseas Governments and Administration,
  St Nicholas House, St Nicholas Road, Sutton, Surrey SM1 1EL.
East European Partnership,
  15 Princeton Court, 53–55 Felsham Road, London SW15 1AZ.
Federation of Recruitment and Employment Services,
  10 Belgrave Square, London SW1X 8PH.
HCA International Ltd,
  49 Wigmore Street, London W1H 9LE.
International Council of Nurses,
  3 Place Jean-Marteau, 1201 Geneva, Switzerland.
International Hospitals Group,
  Stoke Park, Stoke Poges, Slough, Berks SL2 4HS.
International Voluntary Services,
  53 Regent Road, Leicester LE1 6YL.
Overseas Jobs Express,
  PO Box 22 Brighton BN1 6HX.
Overseas Placing Unit,
  Employment Service, PP4 Rockingham House, 123 West Street, Sheffield, West Yorkshire S1 4ER.
Oxfam,
  Oxford House, 274 Banbury Road, Oxford OX2 7DZ.
PGL Young Adventures Ltd,
  Alton Court, Penyard Lane, Ross-on-Wye HR9 5NR.
Raleigh International,
  The Power House, Alpha Place, Flood Street, London SW3 5SZ.
Red Cross,
  9 Grosvenor Cresent, London SW1X 7EJ.

Returned Volunteer Action,
1 Amwell Street, London EC1R 1UL.
Royal College of Nursing International Division,
20 Cavendish Square, London W1M 0AB.
Save the Children Fund,
Mary Datchelor House, 17 Grove Lane, Camberwell, London SE5 8RD.
The Commonwealth Foundation,
Marlborough House, Pall Mall, London SW1Y 5HY.
The Florence and Donald McGregor Trust,
c/o Maurice Plaskow, 9 Lakeside, Oaklands Drive, Weybridge, Surrey.
United National International Service,
3 Whitehall Court, London SW1A 2EL.
Vacation Work,
9 Park End Street, Oxford.
Voluntary Services Overseas,
Enquiries Unit, 9 Belgrave Square, London SW1X 8PW.

12

Private Health Care Opportunities

SCHOOL MATRON

The title carries with it a sometimes stuffy image; in fact, this image is far from reality. Often well loved and in charge of health-related matters in boarding schools or schools that are lucky enough to have their own nurse, the matron is held in high esteem. Entry qualifications, working conditions and pay are entirely dependent upon the employing organization itself. At boarding schools it is not unusual for the job specification to stipulate that the nurse is resident. There is a high degree of responsibility attached to this kind of post since the post holder is often the only medically qualified person on site. This is probably not a job for the inexperienced or those who are afraid of responsibility. The rewards of this type of position include relative independence and the opportunity to develop a service well beyond basic first aid and into preventative health care. Close links with the local general practitioner service could enable many improvements in the service. Vacancies are advertised in the local newspaper, *Times Educational Supplement* or publications such as *The Lady* and *Nursing Times*.

COLLEGE NURSE

Sometimes working alone or as part of a small team the college nurse has the opportunity to extend beyond the basics of first aid by agreement with the employer. Examples of the kind of work undertaken by college nurses include 'look after yourself' programmes for the staff and first aid night classes for fee-paying students. The college nurse may come from a variety of health care settings but accident and emergency experience along with a first aid certificate are very useful. For those who wish to undertake the teaching of first aid as part of the college's activities it will be necessary to undertake a First Aid Course Tutors instruction course. Such courses are run by the Red Cross and St John Ambulance.

Vacancies are advertised in the local press, *Nursing Journal* and *Times Educational Supplement.*

NURSING HOMES AND REST HOMES

Nursing homes and rest homes present a wide variety of opportunities for the qualified nurse, from the chance to give individualized care to partnership prospects. Opportunities vary from home to home and are partly a reflection of the owner/manager's attitudes and partly due to the commitment of the nurses themselves.

Education, training and staff development are areas that many nursing homes and private care homes do not currently address in great depth. Nevertheless most homes would welcome an in-house training programme. The qualified nurse is well placed to develop such a programme. Do not be afraid to ask local experts, such as the MacMillan nurses, to come and talk about their work. In most cases people are willing to talk for nothing or almost nothing, but check this out first. Some aspects of a development programme may include sessions on feeding and nutrition for the nursing assistants, updating the staff on lifting and handling techniques and starting a journal club. Presenting information about practice developments in the nursing press to the other staff could become a regular feature. For some aspects of the programme it may be necessary for the nursing home/care home to send the nurse on a training course/day about the subject itself, but this will be a far more economic way than sending everybody. The benefits of arranging a well-organized programme from which the owners, managers, staff and patients benefit are enormous. Apart from improvements in the quality of care and the respect of the staff, other opportunities can be gained, such as the chance to attend more courses and make contacts with other people. If the staff development course is particularly good, other establishments may wish to send their staff. A small charge could be made for attendance. Try advertising anything you do (with the permission of the owner) that is particularly good or useful. Ensure that any practical procedures (such as lifting and handling, massage) are research-based and meet current legal and professional requirements.

Nursing homes are required to have a first level nurse as the registered nurse in charge but this does not mean that a second level nurse cannot have a financial, administrative or managerial role within the home. Opportunities in the care home/rest home are perhaps slightly different, in that the home does not currently have to be in the name of a registered general nurse. Apart from delivering patient care it may be that the second level nurse could have the opportunity to learn about the mechanics of running a business and a care home. At a later date this may prove useful if the nurse wishes to proceed into management, administration or even partnership/ownership of any health care establishment. Most owners/managers are willing to share information and train employees. It could be that they would be only too pleased to share the workload and this may be an opportunity for promotion within the home or group of homes.

Clinical experts are invaluable to homes of all descriptions. The nurses in post have to carry out a wide range of activities on a daily basis but not many of the nurses are specialists. Homes find it hard to access specialists that larger organizations such as hospitals have: specialist skills that could be of use include those of the continence nurses and diabetes nurse. Many major organizations have specialist nurses who would be only too willing to help the care home nurse develop some of these skills. The Royal College of Nursing has a number of specialist groups such as the RCN Association of Care of the Elderly, the Coronary Heart Disease Forum and the Stoma Care Nursing Forum. Most specialist nurses have study days and regular meetings or forums. The benefits to the home of having a specialist adviser who can help the patients and staff in a problem area such as incontinence is tremendous. While this might not immediately result in promotion or further financial gain for the qualified nurse the amount of job satisfaction to be gained is enormous. Become a resource that will help both you and your patients.

Rehabilitation and mental health nurses have increased job opportunities in the private sector, since much more of this type of nursing is now carried out in the community and private homes. See the section on specialty nursing for details of courses that may be relevant.

Currently, opportunities for advancement are either advertised internally or in the national press. A speculative approach to nursing or care home groups may be advantageous, particularly if the group is expanding and opening new homes. A list of addresses and telephone numbers of the groups and individual homes can be obtained from Social Services departments, who have knowledge of local homes, or the Nursing Homes Association.

PRIVATE HOSPITALS

Many of the opportunities outlined in the Health Services chapter and the nursing home section of this chapter are applicable to the private hospital setting. Progressive private hospital groups are actively trying to lead some nursing developments. BUPA have produced some quality assurance tools which at the time of going to press are extremely progressive. Practice development and personalized quality care are high on the agenda. The hospitals therefore welcome the enthusiastic nurse who is willing and able to advance care. For the nurse who wishes to undertake further study or project work, private hospitals could prove to be very supportive. Some private hospital groups, in common with private nursing home groups, are implementing education and training programmes which include NVQs. For the qualified nurse this provides an opportunity to undertake further training and to teach as part of the training system.

Qualified nurses working within organizations such as Nuffield and BUPA have other training and professional development opportunities. BUPA has appointed a nurse consultant in education and practice to undertake the administration of PREP and develop education and practice within BUPA. Links and joint appointments have been made between BUPA and local colleges of nursing.

With the right training and motivation it could be possible to move into counselling, administration or nursing agency work. Contact the personnel offices of BUPA and Nuffield Hospitals for current opportunities. Some of the more widely advertised jobs appear in the non-NHS sections of nursing journals. A directory of independent hospitals is contained within the *Hospitals and Health Service Yearbook*.

USEFUL READING

Bailey J (1992) Leading from the front. *Nursing Standard*, **6**(19): 20–1.
Chaplain N (ed) (1991) *The Hospital and Health Service Yearbook*. London: Institute of Health Service Management.
Longmans Group (eds) (1992) *Directory of Independent Hospitals and Health Services*. Harlow: Longman.
Schroeder I (1992) Independent women. *Nursing Times*, **88**(4): 79–81.

USEFUL JOURNALS

Nursing Times, Macmillan Magazines, Basingstoke.
Times Educational Supplement, News International plc, London.
The Lady, 39–40 Bedford Street, London WC2E 9ER.

USEFUL ADDRESSES

AMI Healthcare,
    4 Cornwall Terrace, Regents Park, London NW1 4PQ.
BUPA Hospitals,
    Dolphyn Court, Great Turnstile, Lincolns Inn Fields,
    London WC1 7JU.
British Red Cross Society,
    9 Grosvenor Crescent, London SW1X 7EJ.
Community Hospitals plc,
    Sovereign House, 2 Castle Lane, High Street, Bedford MK40 1RY.

Nestor Medical Services,
  15 Southampton Place, London WC1A 2BU.
Nuffield Hospitals,
  Aldwych House, 71–91 Aldwych, London WC2B 4EE.
Nursing Homes Association,
  Calthorpe House, Hagley Road, Edgbaston, Birmingham B16 8QY.
St Andrew's Ambulance,
  16 Torphichen Street, Edinburgh, Scotland EH3 8JB.
St John Ambulance,
  1 Grosvenor Cresent, London SW1X 7EF.

COMPANIES

Many companies now employ occupational health nurses in various
capacities. Larger companies such as water authorities have a number
of occupational health nurses in different capacities. Sometimes nurses
are employed in these departments as part of a team that is delivering
preventative medicine to a large workforce and monitoring conditions
in the workplace. This type of work can be extremely interesting and
could provide avenues into different areas of work within companies,
such as Boots the Chemist and Marks and Spencer plc. Contact the personnel department of major companies and ask for details of vacancies
or even make a speculative move by expressing an interest in their
company and sending details of yourself and the type of work you are
looking for. Details of the major employers in the UK (including banks,
pharmaceutical companies, etc.) are published in a helpful volume called
the *Job Book* (Postle 1992). The volumes *Britain's Privately Owned Companies – the Top 2000* and *Scotland's Top 1000 Companies* are also useful
reading. *Kelly's Directories*, available in most local libraries, provide
details of local companies.

Businesses such as pharmaceutical and health care product companies have some interesting opportunities for enrolled nurses, which
include research nurses, health care trainers, sales representatives
and demonstrators. Many of the major companies have very good
opportunities for promotion and international work for the committed
individual. Once working for the larger companies, personal application
and effort on the job are likely to count for a lot in promotion terms.
The best private companies reward loyalty, effort and results regardless
of qualifications.

Vacancy advertisements can be found in the non-NHS section of the
nursing journals, in newspapers such as the *Guardian* and in other
journals such as *Health Services Journal* and *New Scientist*. Approaching
the well-known nursing agencies or a speculative approach to the companies themselves may have good results.

REFERENCE

Postle J (1992) *The Job Book, 1992.* Cambridge: Hobsons Publishing.

USEFUL READING

Britain's Privately Owned Companies, Vol 1. *Top 2000.* London: Jordan's Business Information Services.

Britain's Privately Owned Companies, Vol 2. *The Next 2000.* London: Jordan's Business Information Services.

Guardian. London: Guardian Newspapers Ltd.

Health Services Journal. London: Macmillan Magazines.

Independent. London: Newspaper Publications.

Kelly's Directories. East Grinstead: Kelly's Directories Ltd.

New Scientist. London: Holborn Publishing.

Scotland's Top 1000 Companies. London: Jordan's Business Information Services.

13

Nursing Agencies

Nursing agencies offer a wide variety of opportunities, many of which do not reach the wider job market. The best agencies look after the nurses that work for them and opportunities for those individuals who work permanently for the agency can be extremely interesting. Often the permanent agency nurse will have priority when the job vacancies come into the office and while the pay may only be at a basic grade it is an opportunity to explore different avenues and to keep many skills alive. Some agencies have long-term contracts with employers and are able to offer nurses who work for them as their main occupation the chance to gain some specialist experience which the nurse may not otherwise gain.

Examples of this include occupational health nursing and research work. In both cases, the inexperienced nurse attempting to find work in either of these fields many find it difficult to get a permanent job with an employer without some previous experience. I have known employers take agency nurses on a temporary basis with little or no experience of either occupational health nursing or research. Opportunities such as these can help the nurse to gain valuable experience for permanent job applications. If you have a particular interest and would like to gain some experience in the discipline, most agencies will try to find you relevant work.

Nursing agencies can be a useful stopgap between main periods of employment. This particular form of 'time out' is useful, because it provides the nurse with the chance to alter hours, working conditions and experiences without taking a career break. Many nurses find new direction after a period of employment with an agency. Some nurses choose agency employment because of the greater flexibility and control that they have over working hours and situations. The good agency nurse is often offered permanent employment by the companies and organizations that they have worked for and who are happy with their services.

Attitudes towards agency nurses are changing. Many employers now recognize that a good agency nurse is a valuable asset. With the ability to adapt easily, to fit into new teams and with a wide variety of skills, the best agency nurses can be moved around with ease, unlike many members of the permanent team. Being an agency nurse whom managers frequently request by name, and a credit to the agency, is a fulfilling career in its own right.

Agencies offer nurses the chance to work on an occasional basis for the occasional shift; many nurses who do this type of work do so in addition to other employment. This type of employment does offer individuals the chance to earn extra money and to gain different experiences; it also, however, requires confidence and stamina on the part of the nurse. Given the small amount of time and type of expertise that the nurse is able to offer the agency the nurse should consider what type of work he/she would be best placed to deliver before accepting any offer of temporary work.

Nursing agencies have details of permanent jobs placed with them as part of their recruitment function. If you are in employment and wish to change your post it can be helpful to register with a reputable large agency with the specific aim of finding another post. It is not necessary to work with the agency in any other capacity in order to use this service. In most cases the employer will pay the agency a fee when the right candidate is found. Check the terms and conditions of the agency's recruitment facility before you register.

In addition to practical nursing opportunities large agencies have a career structure of their own. Most agencies seem to want registered general nurses, but some will employ enrolled nurses as members of the branch staff. Branch staff administer the hundreds of nurses that are booked out into employment and liaise with employers. Other functions include interviewing nurses who wish to work for the agency and visiting employers and clients. Branch staff can move on to management of branch offices and from there to regional management. Large companies such as the British Nursing Association offer some attractive career prospects. The British Nursing Association is part of the multimillion pound international company Nestor.

Because there are a large number of registered nursing agencies be careful to choose a reputable one with whom good employers are likely to want to work. Check the agency's reputation and details before you register. Many nursing agencies are registered with the Federation of Recruitment and Employment Services (FRES) and are listed in the FRES yearbook of recruitment and employment services. Agencies cannot guarantee employment and it is important to remember that once registered as a nurse with an agency the agency usually handles taxation and National Insurance matters, although you are still classed as self-employed. The big agencies are as good as permanent employers and opportunities for the good agency nurse are tremendous. Agencies advertise in most of the main nursing journals and can be found in your local *Yellow Pages*.

USEFUL ADDRESSES

British Nursing Association,
   82 Great North Road, Hatfield, Hertfordshire AL9 5BL.
Federation of Recruitment and Employment Services,
   36–38 Mortimer Street, London W1N 7BB.

14

Opportunities for which Nursing is Useful

THERAPIST

Alternative medicine/therapy is becoming increasingly popular, both within the Health Service and outside it. Aromatherapy and homoeopathy are two such disciplines that can be trained for by part-time study; in the case of homoeopathy there is currently a considerable shortage of practitioners. Entrants into homoeopathy come through one of two routes. For qualified doctors, the homoeopathy course is a short one designed to supplement their training. For all other entrants the course is a full-length one which can be undertaken either in the form of home study with weekend study periods in college, or of formal classes. For further details contact the professional bodies for these disciplines. A general word of advice would be to make sure that any course that you undertake is approved by the professional body and leads to some form of qualification. To undertake any other course would not only be a waste of time but may also result in dangerous practice.

CHILDMINDER

The childminder is playing an increasing role in society and one for which the qualified nurse has some excellent skills. This type of opportunity is particularly useful for the person who wishes to leave nursing and bring up his/her own family, or the individual who would prefer to work independently from home. Childminders must be registered with the local council, who have varying rules and restrictions. Some local colleges offer relevant short courses. Contact your local council for full details of requirements and regulations in your area. Income from childminding is variable.

TEACHER/COACH

Yoga, sports, health and fitness teacher: for all these, nursing is a useful qualification but not the main one. Enthusiasm, experience and qualifications are essential ingredients. Approach the relevant sports body or the Iyengar Institute for further details about training for these opportunities. In most cases teachers/coaches can operate as independent practitioners using school halls, local facilities for classes or they may wish to be affiliated to a local college.

Earnings for highly motivated independent coaches/teachers can be very good.

COUNSELLOR/BEAUTICIAN

Beautician, healthy lifestyle counsellor and many more independent opportunities may be both a sideline and a successful career for the enrolled nurse who wants to change direction but to continue to work in a practical sense with people.

ALEXANDER TECHNIQUE

Some opportunities combine teaching and practice. The Alexander Technique is one such practice. Contact the Society of Teachers of the Alexander Technique for more details.

SOCIAL WORKER

The term 'social worker' covers a wide variety of jobs and skills from the unqualified assistant in a care setting to the highly qualified professional organizing a complete service across a county. There are many openings in social work for which the nursing qualification would be extremely useful.

Social workers run residential homes for the elderly and disabled. They staff and run children's homes, respite centres and family centres. In other instances social workers can be found helping people to meet their housing, financial and other social needs. Some social workers are engaged in fieldwork taking responsibility for a special caseload or particular individuals. Good interpersonal skills are essential for this type of work, which can simultaneously be both frustrating and extremely rewarding. Many social workers are employed directly by local councils or are attached to other large employers such as Health Authorities. Health Authorities employ social workers according to their needs. Large city hospitals will have specialists such as medical social workers who specialize in the elderly; small hospitals may only have one social worker who is attached to the organization. Good local Careers Advisory Services should be able to supply you with details of local opportunities and perhaps even the chance to discuss career prospects with a social worker.

There are three main social work qualifications: the Certificate of Qualification in Social Work (CQSW), which is a mainly college-based course, the Certificate in Social Services (CSS), which is employment-based with some college attendance, and finally the Diploma in Social Work (DipSW), an advanced qualification. Full details of these courses and other training can be obtained from the Central Council for Education and Training in Social Work. The social worker education and training programme is currently trying to incorporate National Vocational Qualifications (NVQ) into the system. With the accreditation of prior learning it may be possible to have nursing qualifications taken into consideration when applying to join the profession. Vacancies and opportunities in social work are advertised in the *Guardian*, local newspapers, *Care Weekly*, *Social Work Today* and *Community Care*.

USEFUL READING

Care Weekly. London: Inside Communication.
Community Care. Sutton: Reed Publishing.
Guardian. London: Guardian Newspapers Ltd.
Maher G (ed) (1990) *Starting a Career in Alternative Medicine.* Kenton: Tackmark Publishing.
Maitland J & Goodliffe H (1989) The Alexander Technique. *Nursing Times*, **85**(42): 54–8.
Social Work Today, **85**(42): Macmillan Magazines, London.

USEFUL ADDRESSES

Central Council for Training in Social Work,
    Derbyshire House, St Chads Street, London WC1H.
National Council for Vocational Qualifications,
    222 Euston Road, London NW1 2B2.
National Institute for Social Work,
    Mary Ward House, 5–7 Tavistock Place, London WC1H 9SS.
Society of Alexander Teachers,
    853 Finchley Road, London NW11 8LX.

15

Opportunities Allied to Nursing

Within the Health Service there are many avenues open to the qualified nurse, a large number of which are not directly related to nursing but for which a nursing qualification or experience would be a great help.

ADMINISTRATION, MANAGEMENT AND SUPPORT ROLES

From time to time opportunities for administration assistants in various departments are advertised within the Health Service and the local press. Qualifications for the jobs are dependent upon the tasks involved; some opportunities have a training programme for new starters, or qualifications which are gained while in post. If you are interested in administration and support posts it would be useful to talk to the Personnel Officer of your local hospital. There are opportunities for administrative assistants to enter the management structure while taking professional qualifications at the same time. Many Health Authorities now offer management open learning certificates and diplomas. A large number offer access to the National Health Services Management Training scheme. Entry for this tends to come from the higher professional and administrative grades, which usually requires 'A' levels as minimum. Local universities and colleges of further education have increasingly more qualifications within their business studies sections that are relevant to Health Service administration and management. The Open University runs a number of courses that are directly relevant and many that may be useful. In the case of the universities and colleges mature students (over 21) may be taken without the necessary entry qualifications provided that the student can prove that he/she is able to cope with the work to the required standard. Ask the particular course tutor or admissions tutor for further details.

Administrative assistants work in personnel departments helping to cope with issues as wide-ranging as training, disciplinary procedures and selection of candidates for jobs in all sections of the Health Service. Other assistants work within departments such as finance, where providing information to help managers make decisions and write reports is vital. In departments that handle equipment and supplies assistants are often responsible for organizing specific activities by themselves and may be responsible for other members of staff.

Management posts that arise are usually advertised both internally and within the *Health Services Journal.* Competition for the junior management posts can be extremely fierce. Management posts that are either trainee or junior usually require the post holders to be undertaking further training towards professional qualifications, e.g. chartered accountancy.

Secretarial and support services, such as clerical, are perhaps the easiest and quickest way to move into the administrative branch. Qualifications and skills for these types of jobs can be easily obtained at night classes. Word processing, desktop publishing and typing skills can be used extensively outside the Health Service; choose a certificated course approved by a well-known body, for example Pitmans. Details of courses available and further information can be obtained from your local further education college.

Far from being a dull option, administration and management offer an ever-increasing number of opportunities for people with a variety of skills and qualifications, the ability to make decisions in an ever-changing environment being an essential qualification. Many people enter into administration and management in order to affect and influence what happens to nursing at a different level. People with particular skills, such as an aptitude for figures or the written word, may find an opportunity to train within a particular niche such as accountancy.

OPPORTUNITIES WITHIN OTHER PROFESSIONS AND DISCIPLINES

Jobs in this section fall into professional and technical/social roles. For many roles fact sheets are available containing details of entry requirements and useful details about the training and development opportunities. These fact sheets can be obtained from the local hospital's personnel department or the local careers office.

TECHNICAL AND SUPPORT ROLES

Technicians are employed in many departments within the local hospitals and community facilities. Roles include artificial kidney technician, audiology, cardiology, neurophysiology and many others. Entry qualifications for these roles range from no GCSEs to four or five. Training and qualifications for the job are gained while in post. Further details about these specific jobs can be obtained from the respective professional bodies. Technicians are also employed in operating theatres; they may be called operating department assistants (ODA). There are no specific entry qualifications for ODAs. The training is gained while in post and leads to the City and Guilds Institute Certificate (a two-year course). In the pharmacy department, technicians are used in the preparation and dispensation of prescriptions. Entry qualifications are normally four GCSEs at least, one of which should be a science. Training is gained over two years while in post and leads to the BTEC Certificate in Pharmaceutical Sciences. Pathology department technicians require no specific entry qualifications but gain qualifications over a two-year period while in post.

Large departments such as linen/laundry services and catering employ management grades with good career prospects. Entry qualifications vary according to the role, but many will take entry at four GCSEs and then release post holders for further study; contact the local personnel officer for more details. For details of opportunities in the Ambulance Service contact your local Health Authority.

For further details about the above opportunities and many more besides ask the local Careers Office/personnel department for the leaflet HSCI (*Health Service Careers*).

PROFESSIONS

Entry to most professions such as physiotherapy, speech therapy, medicine and occupational therapy require a full-time training at college or university lasting from three to five years. Entry for these courses is normally five GCSEs including at least two 'A' levels in relevant subjects. The qualified nurse who has the qualifications should be able to gain direct entry. For the qualified nurse who has almost the right qualifications or who can impress the relevant colleges/universities, it may be possible to gain entry. Ask the particular college/university about mature entry and ask for your qualifications and experience as an enrolled nurse to be taken into consideration. Professions which are fairly closely allied to nursing in which it may be possible to gain entry include physiotherapy, health education and chiropody.

Full details and addresses for all the many opportunities available within the Health Service can be obtained from the manual *Careers in the Health Services* at your local library.

USEFUL READING

Cormack D (ed) (1990) *Developing Your Career in Nursing.* London: Chapman and Hall.

Health Services Journal. London: Macmillan Magazines.

Department of Health (1988) *Health Services Careers.* London: HMSO.

USEFUL ADDRESSES

British Association of Art Therapists,
13c Northwood Road, London N6 5TL.

British Association of Drama Therapists,
PO Box 98, Kirbymoorside, York YO6 6EX.

British Association of Occupational Therapists,
20 Rede Place, Bayswater, London W2 4TU.

British Association of Operating Department Assistants,
Guardian House, 92/94 Foxberry Road, London SE4 2SH.

British Institute of Management,
Management House, Cottingham Road, Corby, Northants NN17 1TT.

Chartered Society of Physiotherapy,
14 Bedford Row, London W1M 8BN.

Cheltenham Tuturial College, 451 High Street, Cheltenham, Glos GL50 3HX.

College of Speech Therapists,
Harold Poster House, 6 Lechmere Road, London NW2 5BU.

Health Education Authority,
Hamilton House, Mabledon Place, London WC1H 9TX.

Health Service Careers,
PO Box 204, London SE5 7ES.

Hotel Services Training Unit,
David Salomons House, Broomhill Road, Southborough, Tunbridge Wells, Kent TN3 0T6.

Institute of Health Services Management,
73 Portland Place, London W1N 4AN.

Institute of Personnel Management,
35 Camp Road, London SW19.

Management Training Scheme,
National Health Service Training Authority, St Bartholomew's Court, 18 Christmas Street, Bristol BS1 5BT.

16

Your Own Business

Starting a small business, working for yourself or in partnership, needs careful planning. In addition to the right qualifications and experience, you will need financial advice and backing, a good business plan and customers. Before you start to work on your own consult a good accountant and bank manager, take advice from the local Business Advisory Service and consult the professional body within which you intend to practise. Membership of a professional organization which provides indemnity insurance is vital.

Most nurses have a wide range of interpersonal skills that will help when starting on their own. Options that are most likely to appeal to nurses who wish to work for themselves in private practice include: Bach flower therapy, chiropractic, dietary therapy, macrobiotics, aromatherapy, homoeopathy, massage, yoga, reflexology, Alexander Technique and counselling.

A particularly useful guide for individuals who are contemplating private practice is the manual/directory of alternative courses *Starting a Career in Alternative Medicine*, edited by G. Maher (1990) and published by Tackmark. This volume lists and describes therapies that include: craniosacral therapy, herbalism, magnetotherapy, iridology, biochemical tissue salts therapy, acupuncture, osteopathy, biomagnetic therapy, auricular therapy, shiatsu, natropathy and many others. The volume also contains details of useful addresses and courses along with some helpful general advice. Many opportunities that are open to qualified nurses can be converted into successful small businesses. Examples of these include counsellor/counselling services, yoga teacher, private office services, baby-sitting agency, dried flower floristry, private teacher and lawyer.

Setting up in private practice can include freelance work. Counselling is perhaps a good example of a private service that can be run with little outlay and produce a reasonable income. Speak to other private practitioners before you begin. Find out about some of the best ways to start and the pitfalls to avoid. Affiliate yourself to the professional organization and undertake only those courses that are recognized by the professions. For most of these ventures there will be regulations for the space that you use and the services that you offer. For instance, agencies must be registered with the local authority under the Agencies Act. Childminders must be registered, their properties must be to a certain standard and their qualifications impeccable. Most professions and trades have unions or professional bodies to which you may have to be affiliated in order to practise. Membership usually has insurance and advice benefits attached. In all respects, treat setting up on your own in private practice as a proper business. Undertake market research and take the right advice before you start.

If you choose to undertake a larger venture such as a nursing home or rest home, contact the local authority for details of local requirements and bodies, such as the Nursing Homes Association, for help and advice. A good bank manager and accountant are essential for larger ventures. In addition to meeting basic requirements for the practical/service aspect of the business you need to have a wide range of business skills. As a self-employed person you need to be a jack of many trades in order to be successful; skills you will need include: marketing, book-keeping, personnel skills (if you employ other people) and boundless energy. Before you begin it is usual to have a business plan; discuss this with someone who is experienced, such as a bank manager. You should carry out some market research to find out if your product is needed, is the right price and in which market you are going to achieve the best results.

The object of this section is not to discuss setting up your own business in depth, but to point out that the person about to set up a small business needs to gain a large number of skills and to have the right product at the right time. Many further education colleges currently run short courses for those who want to start their own businesses. There are many books available in most bookshops which spell out the necessary steps and pitfalls. Advice is available from bank managers, accountants and the Small Business Association. Some of these services have to be paid for; advice from the Small Business Association is usually free and is independent advice. Various advice leaflets ranging from employing people to administering VAT can be obtained from the Inland Revenue and Customs and Excise Offices. *The Lloyds Bank Small Business Guide* by Sara Williams (1987) provides a useful starting handbook.

The rewards from being self-employed can be considerable, a better quality of life and more independence to name but two. On the other hand, the losses can be great, so before you start get plenty of advice and experience. Plan and research the business in great detail.

USEFUL READING

Maher G (ed) (1990) *Starting a Career in Alternative Medicine*. Kenton: Tackmark Publishing.
Williams S (1987) *Lloyds Bank Small Business Guide*. London: Penguin.

USEFUL ADDRESSES

Association of Certified Accountants,
    29 Lincolns Inn Fields, London WC2A 3EE.
Association of Independent Businesses,
    Trowbray House, 108 Weston Street, London SE1.
Association of Reflexologists,
    27 Old Gloucester Street, London WC1N 3XX.
British Acupuncture Association,
    34 Alderney Street, London SW1V 4EV.
British Association for Counselling,
    37a Sheep Street, Rugby, Warwickshire CB21 3BX.
British Chiropractic Association,
    Premier House, 10 Greycoat Place, London SW1P 1SB.
British and European Osteopathic Association,
    6 Adele Road, Teddington, Middlesex.
British Herbal Medicine Association,
    Field House, Lye Hole Lane, Redhill, Avon BS18 7TB.
British Homoeopathic Association,
    27a Devonshire Street, London W1N 1RJ.
British Naturopathic and Osteopathic Association,
    6 Netherhall Gardens, London NW3 5RR.
British Reflexology Association,
    Monks Orchard, Whitbourne, Worcester WR6 5RB.
Faculty of Homoeopathy,
    Royal London Homoeopathic Hospital, Great Ormond Street, London WC1N 3HR.
Highlands and Islands Development Board,
    Bridge House, 27 Bank Street, Inverness IVI 1QR.
Institute of Chartered Accountants in England and Wales,
    Chartered Accountants Hall, PO Box 433, Moorgate Place, London EC2P 2BJ.
Institute of Chartered Accountants of Scotland,
    27 Queen Street, Edinburgh EH2 1LA.
Institute for Complementary Medicine,
    21 Portland Place, London W1N 3AF.
Institute of Management Consultants,
    5th Floor, 32–33 Hatton Garden, London EC1 8DL.

Iyengar Institute,
223a Randolph Avenue, London W9 1NL.
Manpower Services Commission,
Moorfoot, Sheffield S1 4PQ.
National Childminding Association,
8 Masons Hill, Bromley, Kent BR2 9EY.
National Federation of Self Employed and Small Businesses,
32 St Annes Road West, Lytham St Annes, Lancashire FY8 1NY.
Natural Medicine Society,
Regency House, 97–107 Hagley Road, Birmingham B16 8BR.
Nursing Homes Association,
Calthorpe House, Hagley Road, Edgbaston, Birmingham B16 8QY.
Scottish Development Agency,
Small Business Division, Rosebery House, Haymarket Terrace, Edinburgh EH12 5EZ.
Small Firms Centres.
Addresses of local branches are in the telephone directories. Alternatively, telephone 100 and ask for Freefone Enterprise.
The International Federation of Aromatherapists,
Room 8, Department of Continuing Education, The Royal Masonic Hospital, Ravenscourt Park, London W6 0TN.
The Local Enterprise Development Unit,
LEDU House, Upper Galwally, Belfast BT8 4TB.
The Prince's Youth Business Trust,
8 Jockeyfields, London WC1R 4TJ.
The Small Business Bureau,
32 Smith Square, London SW1P 3HH.
Welsh Development Agency,
Head Office, Treforest Industrial Estate, Pontypridd, Mid Glamorgan CF37 5UT.

17

Create your own Opportunities

Qualified nurses who are resourceful can enhance their working lives and professional development by creating their own opportunities. Nearly all the opportunities described elsewhere in this volume are external. To take advantage of these opportunities the nurse has either to make a job move or to undertake some kind of further education that has been created by someone else. Moving from one job to another or undertaking costly courses and education that require considerable energy outside the workplace is not always suitable for every nurse, for a variety of reasons. Nurses in this situation can be very creative without changing their personal and professional circumstances.

The number of initiatives is potentially infinite and limited only by the degree of enthusiasm and energy that is committed to the project. It could be argued that the opportunities that are created within and generated by individuals are the foundations of true nursing development units. Equally, it is probable that nurse consultant status can only be reached by individuals who are capable of this creative process.

PROJECTS AND SPECIALIZATION

Every clinical area, whether it is in the public or private sector, primary or secondary care has need of specialists. Become a specialist who attracts attention from both inside and outside the workplace. Subjects such as incontinence, pressure area care, wound care, dealing with confused patients and counselling are just a few examples. Research the subject, undertake specialist training and study days. Join the relevant special interest groups and make links with other individuals who will be able to help you. Know the companies that supply relevant products. Collect and keep up-to-date information about products, their usage and cost. Be able to plan care accordingly and to help others to do so. Be aware of the professional and legal implications of such a venture and have the support of your manager. If you wish to develop the specialization into an additional service, acquire some teaching and presentation skills, learn how to produce information booklets, packs and leaflets.

FUNDRAISING AND FINANCE

Dynamic individuals may choose to create opportunities of a different kind to the practice-based specialist skills acquiring skills that are not immediately relevant to the workplace but that are useful can be both beneficial to the organization and the individual. Fundraising and finding finance for various projects including education is in effect a small business. Many lessons can be learnt from a one-off fundraising event such as a bed push, but the ongoing long-term programme of income generation is one that requires many skills. Apart from the Open University Winning Resources and Support course there are no formal education programmes that will help you to learn these skills. A friendly charity or voluntary organization may be willing to help you understand some of the processes and ways of making a programme more effective. The Directory of Social Change publish a number of useful volumes which include *The Complete Fundraising Handbook* and *Finding Sponsors*. Having the skills and contacts to be able to raise money for a variety of things can have considerable benefits. Most organizations and individuals are looking for extra finance to help them to improve their current situation for a variety of reasons. A person that acts as a resource and helps them to find money could prove to be invaluable.

PUBLISHING

Publishing has become increasingly more important to nurses over the past decade. Skills ranging from the ability to be able to produce a small polished article for a journal to being an editor or producing your own publication are extremely useful. In-house newsletters are a particularly good example of using small home publishing kits to improve communication between staff, act as a forum for new ideas and enthuse people. In-house newsletters have a habit of going beyond the immediate setting and can help people to understand your organization a little better. A number of colleges now run short courses in home publishing and most publishing houses provide details for would-be authors. The information varies from short notes for contributors to journals to small handbooks/packages for the author of books. The leading journals, such as *Nursing Standard, Nursing Times* and *Health Services Journal,* print details within the regular journals for contributors of articles. *Writing for Nursing and Allied Professions* by Cormack (1984) contains a very concise introduction to the subject of nursing publishing.

STUDIES AND RESEARCH

Special studies and research can be considered an opportunity to acquire new knowledge and skills while contributing to the organization. Effective research applied to practice can be a catalyst for practice and the research worker. Being able to quantify situations and act upon the information is extremely powerful. Using research as a basis for strengthened argument (facts, not theories!) helps organizations and individuals to gain resources and shape practice. Acquiring the relevant skills and using them in the workplace could have tremendous benefits. Research and other projects need to conform to certain guidelines and to take into account ethical issues. Management support should be enlisted for the piece of work.

Not all opportunities need to be one individual's efforts primarily. Determining that your efforts combined with those of others will create a centre of excellence can be a pleasurable challenge. This kind of self-generated opportunity lies in persuading others to join in, enlisting them and effectively harnessing and leading that enthusiasm. Leadership skills are essential for this type of venture. It is important to note that to be able to lead this type of venture properly you do not have to be the immediate manager/sister/charge nurse, but you do have to gain their support, commitment and enthusiasm. Most managers would be happy to let you lead a project if it was managed effectively. Examples of projects that could be led effectively within a motivated team include the introduction of activity nursing, individualized patient care that is a role model for other areas. In care homes, setting up patient-run services such as a small shop and library may be motivating to staff who want to offer new patient-controlled services and motivation to patients who have limited outside activities.

Grasping an initiative before it becomes an order can sometimes turn a chore into an opportunity. Quality assurance, standard setting and audit are good current examples of this process. Inevitably, auditors of care will want to see user-friendly tools and systems that they understand; if not already in place there is a danger that these will be imposed. Why wait until you have to do it? Design a system that is right for you, reflects your care and involves others in the workplace. See if others will undertake part of the project and motivate them to feel good about the inevitable.

REFERENCE

Cormack D (1984) *Writing for Nursing and Allied Professions.* Oxford: Blackwell.

USEFUL READING

Clarke S (1992) *The Complete Fundraising Handbook.* London: Directory of Social Change.

Eastwood M & Casson D (1992) *The Educational Grants Directory,* 2nd edn. London: Directory of Social Change.

Norton M (1989) *How to Write Better Fundraising Applications.* London: Directory of Social Change.

USEFUL ADDRESSES

Directory of Social Change,
Radius Works, Back Lane, London NW3 1HL.
Open University Business School,
Open University, Walton Hall, Milton Keynes MK7 6AA.
Royal College of Nursing (Special Interest Groups)
20 Cavendish Square, London W1M 0AB.

18

Complete Change

Sometimes a completely new direction is the direction of choice. In nearly all cases some form of re-training or further education is required. Many opportunities may be usefully combined with nursing if you wish to continue within the health care setting but in a different capacity. Other opportunities and training may take you into a completely new profession; many of the qualifications required can be gained while you are in your current post. Examples include the following.

Teaching BEd Hons Degree (in-service)

Many institutions now offer a teaching degree for which one can study part-time. Entry qualifications vary, but it mainly depends upon experience. If you can prove conclusively that you are actively involved in teaching/training and are capable of undertaking the course content, approach your local university for further details or consult the handbooks available at your local library. Once again, this qualification could be used to start a career within the education service, Health Service training or private schools. For more details about prospects within education contact 'Teaching as a Second Career' Division at the Department of Education.

Law Degrees

A number of universities are currently offering a part-time degree in law. The course is usually five years long, at the end of which the successful candidate can consider entry into the legal profession and the practical part of a solicitor's qualification. As a degree in its own right this could prove most useful, combined with nursing experience and qualifications. In an era of ever-increasing claims for medical negligence, people with legal qualifications and nursing experience are highly employable both within the management and legal departments of the Health Service and within private practice specializing in medical claims or acting as advisers.

Entry qualifications for the part-time courses vary from institution to institution. For the enrolled nurse without the minimum qualifications an Access course run by the local college (part-time) will give you the relevant entry qualifications and insight into the degree course.

Management

The BTEC HNC Business and Finance course, BTEC HND Computer Studies and the Management Sciences Certificate by Distance Learning and Flexi-study currently run by many universities and colleges are all examples of courses for which entry for mature candidates over twenty-one without the minimum qualifications will be considered on an individual basis. If you are interested in moving into the business world contact the local university or the Open University for relevant courses. Similar qualifications and entry conditions are available in the fields of information/computer studies, leisure studies, accounting and estate agency.

Not everyone wanting to change direction will wish to undertake major study courses in order to move on. Many individuals choose to develop skills that they already have or intend to acquire and generate an income from these.

Design and fashion, printing and textiles

Although fiercely competitive, there are opportunities for those who have flair to undertake evening classes or self-study in order to improve or gain skills. Opportunities resulting from this include private dressmaker and designer, fabric design for small projects and printing on a small scale. For people who want the security of a career or working for a company many useful addresses and contacts, including job advertisements, can be found in the journal *D.R. The Fashion Business* available from most good newsagents.

Desktop publishing/printing

A large number of further education colleges offer short courses in desktop publishing and printing techniques. Before you embark upon the expense of purchasing the relevant equipment it may be worthwhile undertaking a short course and avoiding the pitfalls.

A number of people are able to run successful small businesses printing CVs, publishing short documents and printing business cards. Some people embark upon home printing techniques such as screen printing that will enable them to produce reasonable greetings cards, book-marks, carrier bags, etc.

Arts and crafts

Generally, it is fairly hard to make a living from arts and crafts. Unless you have exceptional ability and flair, or run a fairly aggressive small pottery, you are unlikely to make a substantial living. Some people combine these practical skills with teaching or catering/hotelier activities. Ventures like this include special interest breaks run as a joint project with local bed and breakfast/hotel establishments. Lecture tours or private classes in local halls are popular. A serious business such as a full-time pottery will need to combine not only practical skills but good marketing and management skills and the right outlets.

If you are looking for ideas, visit you next local arts and crafts sale. Purchase one of the many magazines that are sold both at fairs and in the local newsagents. These magazines will have details of suppliers, events and buyers as well as regular features about particular skills.

A word of caution: it is probably not advisable to invest a great deal of money or leave employment for a change of direction into arts and crafts until you have a well-established business that can support you and still be profitable.

Working for others

Needless to say, the numbers of avenues open to you are boundless. A good careers handbook available from newsagents/bookshops or the local library will spell out some of the options. In practice, at a time of high unemployment it may be more difficult to move into a different area. If you are contemplating moving into a completely different line of work it would be useful to gain some practical experience and make a start on acquiring necessary qualifications before you begin to apply.

Many applications fail because the applicant has insufficient experience. Hunt out firms that may be willing to give you occasional employment within the field that you wish to be. If this tactic fails volunteer your services in some capacity or another. Most employing personnel officers are extremely helpful and will point you in the right direction if they cannot help you themselves. For those people who manage to find an occasional employer, if the opportunity arises the firm often takes the individual into full-time employment. In some instances you may have to be prepared to start fairly low on the scale for a short while in order to work your way up to the position you would like to be in. Examples of employers who have good career prospects for different people who come in at all levels include Banks, Building Societies, Marks and Spencer, Trust House Forte and McDonalds.

Some of these businesses have benefits which help to counteract initial loss in salary. For example, building society employees enjoy low mortgage interest rates; some banks have similar deals. Marks and Spencer have a range of subsidized facilities which help offset the cost of living for employees.

Small, new businesses are particularly vulnerable during economic recession. If you choose to take another job within the small business sector the rewards could be very high if you help a business to succeed; on the other hand, if the business fails you may have to find alternative employment. If you choose this option make sure that you have other employment available should this happen.

The publication *Independent Careers*, edited by Boehm and Spalding (1991), contains some particularly useful ideas and contacts for people who wish to work on their own or independently for others.

USEFUL READING

Boehm K & Spalding J L (eds) (1991) *Independent Careers.* London: Bloomsbury.
Burston D (ed) (1991) *A–Z of Careers and Jobs,* 4th edn. London: Kogan Page.
Elsom D & Percival K (eds) (1990) *Job Book 1990.* Cambridge: Hobson.

USEFUL JOURNALS

D.R. The Fashion Business. London: International Thompson Publishing.
Times Educational Supplement. London: News International plc.

USEFUL DIRECTORIES

Benn's Media Directories, 141st edn. Tonbridge: Benn's Media.
Jordan's Directories. Bristol: Jordan's Information Services.
Kelly's Business Directories. East Grinstead: Kelly's Directories.
Britain's Privately Owned Companies, Vols 1 and 2. Bristol: Jordan's Information Services.
Wales Business Directory.

USEFUL ADDRESSES

British Dental Association,
64 Wimpole Street, London W1M 8AL.
BTEC Information Services,

Central House, Upper Woburn Place, London WC1H 0HH.
British Veterinary Association,
  7 Mansfield Street, London W1A 0AT.
Institute of Legal Executives,
  Kempston Manor, Kempston, Bedford MK42 7AB.
Law Society,
  113 Chancery Lane, London WC2A 1PL.
Open University,
  Walton Hall, Milton Keynes MK7 6AA.
Teaching as a Second Career,
  Department of Education, Elizabeth House, York Road, London SE7
  7PH.

Section Three
Towards the Opportunities

1

Training and Education

Qualifications can be broadly categorized into three groups.

- academic qualifications
- vocational qualifications
- experience.

On some occasions the right qualifications may include other, less quantifiable items, such as attitude, ability and potential. It is worth considering qualifications in the widest sense, since employers are often looking not only for formal qualifications and experience, but also the right attitude and potential, for example. If you are contemplating opportunities in a self-employed capacity or working independently within a company, it is essential to have an in-depth understanding of your personal qualities as qualifications for the new role.

ACADEMIC QUALIFICATIONS

Academic qualifications are perhaps the easiest to understand. They have a clearly defined hierarchy from GCSE to Doctor of Philosophy. Each of the levels represents levels of attainment and suggests a degree of subject knowledge. The qualifications are transferable in a way that currently vocational qualifications are not. The system is well established and from an employer's point of view the easiest to use when deciding upon qualifications for the job. Academic qualifications do not indicate the person's ability to make things happen in practice.

VOCATIONAL QUALIFICATIONS

Qualifications such as the Certificate of Qualification in Social Work or the City and Guilds 730 certificate (teaching and presentation) are directly related to specific forms of practice. These and other vocational qualifications have a recognized level within their professions. It is, however, difficult to assess what they are worth compared with each other; this issue is currently being addressed by the National Vocational Council for Qualifications.

EXPERIENCE

Perhaps the most difficult to assess in terms of level and comparison, experience is a key qualification. Two people holding the same grade of job and title may have completely different experiences. It is useful to consider the type and quality of experience that you have had and be able to present this information to potential employers in a manageable form. For future reference many people keep a record of their work experience. The record usually contains details of the following.

- Type of work undertaken.
- Length of employment.
- Full-time/part-time, etc.
- Special skills gained/required while in post.
- Projects/change that you have been involved in.
- Special responsibilities, e.g. management of people, equipment/ stock.
- Contributions to the job in addition to the basic requirements of the post.
- Further training/courses attended while in post.

Details such as these are also kept within the professional profile.

At a later date records like this can be used to quote specific evidence to potential employers that you have the relevant skills and experience. It is easy to forget the details or even the amount and type of different experiences that you have gained over a period of time.

With the exception of an academic qualification, all other qualifications are very difficult to measure up against each other or count towards a higher qualification. For people with a professional vocational qualification such as nursing, this can present a problem if they want to move out into another area of work. If you are considering further education of any description or a change of direction, it may be prudent to choose systems of study, experience or training that are flexible enough to allow you to move again if you have to. It is useful to choose systems that can be added to at a later date and whose qualifications can be compared with other qualifications.

Two such systems that will help you progress without channelling your options are the Open University Academic System and the National

Vocational Qualification Schemes. On a local basis you may find that universities offer a modular approach to study at your own pace. For many higher education courses, there are often linked Access courses run by the local further education colleges.

The English National Board is currently implementing a Credit and Accumulation Transfer System (CATS). A number of its certificated courses have been given credit ratings. A list of courses with credit ratings can be obtained from the English National Board's Learning Resources Centre. A working party comprising the English National Board and the Council for Education and Training in Social Work is currently looking at joint validation of courses.

In all the instances mentioned above you can find your way into these systems without any formal qualifications and work your way into another profession, or gain a qualification such as a degree. Using the systems mentioned above you can approach a new opportunity and gain the relevant qualifications at a pace that suits you without having to move into full-time study.

Increasingly, institutions such as universities are using the accreditation of prior and experiential learning as part of their system. Candidates with particular experience or education can have the length and content of the intended course reduced. This is done on an individual basis by negotiation. Ask the course tutor for more details before you enrol.

ASSESSMENT OF PRIOR EXPERIENTIAL LEARNING (APEL)

Assessment of prior experiential learning (APEL) is a process by which previous experience and learning can be taken into account and used as credit towards another qualification. The amount of credit that you will be given for your prior learning depends upon its relevance to the qualification that you seek. The experience and learning may be practical, skill-based, work-based or life experience and not necessarily formal study. The experience must be clearly identified and capable of being assessed and credit rated. Each application for accreditation is assessed on an individual basis. Colleges and universities are currently developing systems to facilitate the assessment of prior learning.

National Vocational Qualifications have the accreditation of prior experience and learning as a formal part of the system. So for example, a nursing auxiliary could have his/her experience counted towards the qualification of operating department assistant if he/she so wished. It is the intention of the current education system and the Council for Vocational Qualification that in future all professional qualifications will be a part of this system.

International Therapy Examination Council (ITEC) is a system of qualification through which you can gain entry into a number of practical opportunities ranging from beautician to aromatherapy and massage. The courses have modules which, if relevant, can be used towards another ITEC course at a later date.

The qualifications have the added advantage of entitling the holder to membership of a professional association with the benefit of public indemnity insurance. ITEC qualifications are recognized in Japan, America, New Zealand, Australia, India and more than twenty other countries in the world. ITEC now offer an Honours Diploma for excellence. For details of the types and availability of courses contact ITEC.

FRAMEWORK AND HIGHER AWARD

The English National Board's Framework and Higher Award complements PREP and is available to practitioners on the UKCC register with patient contact. The framework is the system within which the practitioner's professional development takes place and leads towards the Higher Award. Development through the framework attracts credit accumulation and transfer ratings; ten key characteristics must be met at the required standard. These key characteristics can be obtained by a number of means, including open learning and inservice training. Individuals enrolled on the Framework and Higher Award scheme are required to maintain a professional portfolio supplied as part of the project. Further details of the Framework and Higher Award can be obtained from the English National Board or local colleges of nursing and professional development units that are facilitating the scheme.

ACCESS COURSES

These courses are a year or two years long on a part-time or full-time basis and are modular. Students select from units of study such as health sciences, social studies, business and information technology and media studies. The course, which contains a number of extended essays and final examinations, may be used as entry to professional training such as physiotherapy, radiography or as access to university. For full details of Access courses available locally and opportunities for successful students, contact the local further education college. Access courses are considered to be tuition to 'A' level standard and are only available to candidates over twenty-one years of age.

The Business and Technical Education Council (BTEC) offer a number of modular courses. These courses are run on a day release, full-time, sandwich, block release and part-time basis. Open and distance learning programmes are also available through BTEC in conjunction with City and Guilds. BTEC offer a number of vocational and pre-vocational courses; the system is one of certificates and diplomas at a national and higher national level. Entry to professional courses such as physiotherapy and degree courses can be gained by a number of options using the BTEC system; contact BTEC Information Services for full details of the courses and availability. Alternatively, contact any of the local colleges and universities currently offering BTEC courses.

CREDIT ACCUMULATION AND TRANSFER SCHEMES (CATS)

Credit Accumulation and Transfer Schemes (CATS) take prior academic study into account as credit towards academic awards. CATS has three main parts: credit accumulation, in which credit for learning is given as it takes place; credit transfer, a system which enables individuals to transfer credits from one career path to another or between institutions; and credit exemption, a reduction in course length or exemption from some aspects of a new course, enabled by taking prior relevant learning into account. CATS has three levels. Level one is worth 120 credits and is certificate level (or the first year of a degree course). Level two is worth 120 credits and is diploma level (or the second year of a degree course). Level three is worth 120 credits and is the third year of a degree.

In common with the vocational qualifications assessment system APEL, the universities and colleges that are adopting CATS are currently evolving systems to administer the necessary individual assessments.

Because there are now a number of routes through which to enter a new occupation, change direction or move to a higher level it is worth examining the system itself to see if:

(a) it will give you credit for your current qualifications and experience, and

(b) you can transfer and use at a higher level any qualifications you may wish to take in the future.

Training and education for the purpose of professional development can be obtained from a number of sources. The most immediate sources are usually the in-house education, training and development programmes run by most good employers. Nurses who want to develop themselves beyond in-house programmes can almost always access a continuing education department, usually attached to a college of nursing. Continuing education departments offer a range of courses designed to meet local needs and many departments offer National Board courses. The courses run by continuing education departments are not just for health service employees; many departments offer places to nurses working in the private health care sector, the Services and other situations. Contact your local department for further details. Many private hospital and nursing home groups have professional development programmes. BUPA now has a professional development adviser.

Many universities now have a comprehensive health services programme with courses that are open to qualified nurses working in all types of situations. Most universities are currently rating their courses on the CATS scheme. Some universities have approved and given CATS ratings to training programmes being run by private companies. One such arrangement exists between Hewlett Packard Ltd Healthcare Education Services and a university. Courses currently being run include Introduction to Ultrasound Technology and Basic ECG Technology.

The Royal College of Nursing Institute of Advanced Studies offers a wide range of courses, some of which are available to enrolled nurses. A comprehensive prospectus can be obtained from the College.

The Open University has a complete department devoted to health studies and offers a wide range of courses from the short course study packs such as the P553 *A Systematic Approach to Nursing Care* to diplomas and degrees. Increasingly, more institutions are offering health care studies on an open learning basis.

USEFUL READING

Kogan Page (1991) *British Qualifications.* London: Kogan Page.
McManus M (1991) Credit accumulation and transfer schemes. *Nursing Standard*, 6(6): 28–30.
Thorne P (1991) Assessment of prior learning. *Nursing Standard*, 6(10): 32–4.
Wells J (1990) *The Directory of Continuing Education and Training for Nurses.* London: Newpoint.

USEFUL ADDRESSES

Birmingham Open Learning Development Unit,
   East Birmingham College, Garrets Green Lane, Birmingham
   B33 0TS.
British Technical Education Council (BTEC),
   Information Services, Central House, Upper Woburn Place, London
   WC1H 0HH.
Cheltenham Tutorial College, 451 High Street, Cheltenham, Glos
   GL50 3HX.

City and Guilds,
  326 City Road, London EC1V 2PT.
Continuing Education,
  Open University, Walton Hall, Milton Keynes MK7 6AA.
Continuing Nurse Education Programme,
  Barnet College, Russell Lane, Whetstone, London N20 0AX.
Distance Learning Centre,
  South Bank University, South Bank Technopark, 90 London Road,
  London SE1 6LN.
English National Board Open Learning Database,
  PO Box 356, Sheffield S8 0SJ.
Hampshire Open Learning Unit,
  PO Box 64, Winchester, Hampshire SO23 8XY.
ITEC,
  James House, Oakelbrook Mill, Newent, Gloucestershire
  GL18 1HG.
National Extension College,
  18 Brooklands Avenue, Cambridge CB2 2HN.
National Council for Vocational Qualifications,
  222 Euston Road, London NW1 2B2.
Open Business School,
  Open University, Walton Hall, Milton Keynes MK7 6AA.
Perth College of Further Education,
  Braham House, Crieff Road, Perth, Scotland PH1 2NX.
Rapid Results College,
  Tuition House, 27–37 St Georges Road, London SW19 4DS.
Royal College of Nursing Institute of Advanced Studies,
  20 Cavendish Square, London W1M 0AB.
SCOTTSU International,
  Northern College of Education, Gadyne Road, Broughty Ferry,
  Dundee DD5 1NY.
Scottish Open Learning Consortium,
  West Lothian College, Lammermuir House, Livingston, Scotland.
The Open College in Lothian,
  24 Milton Road East, Edinburgh EH15 2PP.
The Open College (Manchester),
  Suite 470, St James Building, Oxford Street, Manchester M1 6FQ.
University of London (Department of Extramural Studies),
  Senate House, Malet Street, London WC1E 7HU.

2

Keep Your Options Open

A recent British Institute of Management report, *The Future of Middle Management* (Wheatley 1992), suggests that middle management will need to be able to adapt to continuous change, increased workload and be multi-skilled. In addition to this the middle manager will need to constantly update, be flexible and consider career direction change in the light of increasing redundancies. This is sound advice not only for middle managers, but for all working individuals in an increasingly more competitive environment. Within the profession of nursing the last two years have seen the introduction of a new form of nurse training, P2000, the Post Registration Education and Practice project (PREP) (UKCC 1990) proposals and many local initiatives. It is worth considering that all of this could be developed and changed again. If you are considering embarking upon a further course of training, education or change of direction keep your options open. Choose avenues of study that will enable you to change direction if you have to, or that will give you extra/new skills and continue into the future. If you choose to move out of nursing into a different occupation keep your nursing skills alive, register with an agency or a nurse bank and retain your registration with the UKCC. Attend study/training sessions that will help towards your re-registration. If you embark upon a course of action that does not lead to direct entry into a specific occupation, e.g. self-employed homoeopath or qualified physiotherapist, make sure that the course of action has a number of possible outcomes just in case:

(a) you decide not to enter the new occupation, or
(b) the particular occupation requirements are changed and you have to re-train.

If you choose to move from a more secure occupation such as from nursing within a hospital with a full-time contract to being self-employed make sure that you are able to boost your income if you have to do so.

REFERENCES

Wheatley M (1990) *The Future of Middle Management.* Corby: British Institute of Management.

UKCC (1990) *The Report of the Post Registration Education and Practice Project.* London: UKCC.

3

Changing Your Job

Analyse the reasons for changing your job before you take the step. Take advice from mentors or others who are willing to help you decide which direction to take. Having identified motives and direction begin the search for the particular opportunity that interests you. For those individuals changing their jobs within the profession, the most obvious place to find the right job is within the classified sections of good nursing journals. Opportunities are also advertised on the noticeboards within hospitals and organizations. Nursing agencies have a large number of vacancies of different types, many of which do not reach the nursing press, and are advertised on noticeboards, etc. If you have a specific type of post in mind or a particular place in which you wish to work it is worth consulting the local nursing agencies in addition to the normal routes. If the post that you would like is not advertised it is sometimes worth writing to the employing manager and asking for an informal discussion about opportunities that may occur in the future. Most managers are quite willing to discuss possible opportunities, particularly in larger authorities where there is a fairly frequent turnover of staff and advertising is a constant expense.

If you choose to take the initiative and contact potential employers directly remember that your first telephone call or letter will determine the degree of your success. Research the organization and approach the correct individual using their full title and correct name. Be specific about the nature of your enquiry and concise but not terse in communication. If you make a telephone call be prepared to answer questions about yourself. Have available a list of jobs/tasks that you have done that are relevant to the post you are interested in. Have a copy of your CV on hand.

Because such a large number of interesting jobs do not reach the wider market it may be worth advertising yourself, particularly if you have specialist skills. The back pages of most reputable nursing journals have advertisement sections.

4

Changing Your Career

Changing your job within nursing is a relatively straightforward process. This is not always the case when you try to change your career. Obtaining the first job in a new career will be the most difficult job to get. Before you embark upon the change make sure that you have the relevant qualifications to the correct level of attainment and ideally have gained some experience of the job/profession itself, at least on a voluntary basis. Changing your career begins long before the first job application, even before you acquire the relevant qualifications. Try to gain some practical insight into the new job. Research the type of employers who may be interested in your skills. Identify and undertake courses that are recognized and transferable. Investigate the long-term prospects of the change and future career paths. Be clear about why you want to change your career.

At the time of interview most employers will want to see not only qualifications and commitment from you but a clear understanding of what the new career will involve. Not all employers are enthusiastic about employing people who have changed direction; some may even see this as a disadvantage. Counter any doubts this employer may have by presenting the move in a positive light. Point out that you enjoyed the past career but want to develop in another direction and advance the new career with the skills that may be common to both and the benefits that you could have for the organization as a multi-skilled person. Whatever your new career, the high levels of interpersonal skills and decision making required at all levels of nursing are going to be useful to any organization.

5

Applications

Applications for posts are usually either by application form or curriculum vitae (CV). The method of application is usually indicated in the advertisement by the agency or by the personal contact.

Application forms are obtained by telephone call or letter. In each case keep the contact brief and clear. Give the relevant person your full name and address. Ask for full details in addition to the application form. If you write for an application form remember that the letter will be kept on file, therefore make sure that it is legible, dated, articulate and clearly addressed. Upon receipt of the application form make sure that you are able to complete and return it before the closing date. If there is no closing date return it within two weeks. Before you complete the form photocopy it and use the copy to draft the final application. Read the job description and details in depth. Analyse your own skills and experiences. Match them up to the qualities and qualifications required. Highlight particular pieces of evidence of past work that will enable you to undertake the new post. If you lack particular skills required, investigate ways of acquiring them. Be prepared to answer questions about skill deficit during the interview. Check the salary and conditions of employment, along with details of the organization/employer. Read carefully the information regarding the skills, qualifications, experience and particular attributes that the post requires. Check that you are able to meet the requirements.

Detail personal information, education and career moves to date in the relevant sections and make sure that any career breaks or breaks in education/training are clearly accounted for. Using the photocopy of the application form complete a draft copy making sure that all your experiences are accounted for. Follow the instructions carefully, do not attempt to cram too much onto the form, continue on another piece of paper if necessary.

Some application forms have sections that ask you to detail your current responsibilities. Pay particular reference to those that match up to the responsibilities required in the new job description. Most application forms have a section that asks you for any additional information, special interests, comments in support of your application. This is the section that helps the employer choose between similar candidates. It is your chance to persuade the would-be employer. Describe particular projects, experiences that you have had, led or initiated that are relevant to the job and demonstrate the required skills. Detail interests that are relevant to show specific characteristics. Make sure that this section is grammatically correct, that it flows, is relevant and interesting. Do not boast or include irrelevant material. Draft and re-draft this section, setting it out clearly until you are satisfied.

Type your application form, make sure that it is neat, concise, clear and easy to read. It should be free from spelling mistakes and grammatical errors. Get someone to check it for you. Make sure that your referees are current or fairly recent employers and that you have their permission to give their names as referees. Some referees like to have a copy of the job description for the post you have applied for; it helps the referee make sure that the reference is relevant to the job.

Finally, keep a copy of the completed application form for reference purposes.

CURRICULUM VITAE (CV)

It is useful to keep an up-to-date standard curriculum vitae (CV) ready for the right opportunity. The CV can then be adapted to meet the requirements of the post for which you are applying. Writing a CV from scratch can take up to two days; once you have produced one keep it up to date for future occasions. It is essential to present your career history as clearly and attractively as possible and to decide upon the presentation before the content. All CVs have a section at the top listing biographical details such as name, date of birth, address and next of kin. After the biographical details come details of your education and jobs to date. The layout of these sections is a matter of personal choice. Some people list their education separately from their career experiences, others list education and career together chronologically (see Appendix 1 for an example). In either case, it is essential that the sequence of events is clear, dates are accurate and that the reader is able to get the relevant information quickly. Do not attempt to cram too much into each section. Employers are less likely to be attracted to a candidate whose CV is confusing and time consuming. Detail the experiences and the skills that you have gained which are relevant to the post for which you are applying. If you have not written a CV before look at some examples before you design your own. Some high street typing services or businesses that advertise in the nursing press will be able to help you design a CV; it may be more cost effective for you to have one produced professionally and update and adapt it for later usage. Before you send off a CV check the spelling, content and presentation. Keep a copy.

COVERING LETTER

Most application forms or CVs are accompanied by a covering letter. Keep the letter simple and clear, and if possible type it. It should be clearly addressed to the relevant individual, dated and presented on plain paper of a good quality. It is perfectly acceptable to support your application by including details of a particular skill, experience that you have which is relevant to the post and that would make you suitable for the job. If you are writing to a potential employer who has not advertised a job, enclose your CV and use the covering letter to sell yourself. Acknowledge that there might not be a current vacancy but gratefully request that your letter and CV be kept on file. Do not use a standard letter (every employer will be looking for people who are particularly interested in both the job and the organization). Do not use abbreviations or jargon.

USEFUL READING

Skeats J (1989) *CVs and Written Applications.* London: Ward Lock.

6

Interviews

Before you attend an interview ask someone with interviewing experience to give you some practical help in the form of advice or mock interviews. Draw up a pre-interview checklist using the job description as a framework if possible (see Appendix 2 for an example of a pre-interview checklist).

INFORMAL INTERVIEWS

Informal interviews are sometimes offered to prospective candidates. This is not necessarily an indication that the candidate will be shortlisted. Employers often offer informal interviews as a two-way process. It gives the candidate the opportunity to view the organization and role before application and will help the interviewer decide whether to shortlist or not. Some organizations expect applicants to be interested enough in the organization and job to attend the informal interview, and do not shortlist candidates with insufficient interest, while others offer the interview as a fact-finding exercise and non-attendance will not prejudice the application. In either case, the informal interview is the first face to face contact and the impression created is crucial. Research the organization, know the scale of the operation, the nature of the business and its specialties. Know the interviewer by name, show interest in the job, people and organization. Ask questions that will help you to prepare for the formal interview. Be prepared to answer a few questions about yourself; it is not usual or necessary at this stage to discuss your entire career history. In all other respects treat the informal interview as you would the formal one. Arrive ten minutes early. Wear smart, comfortable clothing. Do not bring excessive amounts of paraphernalia such as briefcases and umbrellas.

FORMAL INTERVIEWS

Perhaps the most intimidating part of the application process is the formal interview. Arrive early. Relax, read through your written application again as you wait to be interviewed. When called into the interview room smile and shake hands with the interviewers. Remember their names once you have been introduced. During the interview answer their questions concisely, giving full details of experience and information asked for without waffling. Make sure that you understand the question before you answer it. Ask them to repeat the question if necessary. Having researched the organization and analysed your own experiences and skills against the job description, you should be able to answer their questions giving examples that demonstrate your competencies. If you are unskilled in a particular area say so, but add that you intend to undertake the necessary training. Express your views and thoughts clearly. Show enthusiasm, do not be evasive and above all do not criticize your current employer. Smile and be pleasant, be positive about yourself and your future. Be sure about how (in cooperation with others) you would undertake the job. If you are asked about strengths and weaknesses do not choose a weakness that is directly related to the job; with every weakness you choose say what you are doing to conquer it. Strengths should be things that are personal qualities or related to the job; do not boast. At the end of the interview it is usual for the candidate to be asked if they have any questions. Do not ask questions that reveal your ignorance of the organization or job, concentrate on development issues such as their vision of the job/organization in two years' time. If all of the issues have been covered and you have no questions do not feel that you have to ask questions. At the close of the interview thank the interviewers.

If you are unsuccessful at interview ask for some feedback. Try to analyse why yourself. Invariably, the interviewers have a list of requirements which include aspects such as the right personality for the team; you may just have been unlucky.

USEFUL READING

Cole A (1989) The other side of the table. *Nursing Times*, **85**(21): 32–4.
Fardell J (1989) Just the job. *Nursing Times*, **85**(21): 27–30.
Stevens M (1989) *Winning at your Interview*. London: Kogan Page.

7

Career Mentorship

Perhaps the greatest help that you can receive while you are planning the future is the help of a mentor. If you work in a setting where mentorship is not a part of the system seek to identify your own mentor.

A mentor is someone who takes a personal interest in your development, guides and supports you, somebody whom you respect as a person and a professional. If the organization in which you work does not have a mentorship system find your own mentor. Most people are happy to be approached and to offer their support. Choose your mentor with care. Make sure that they have enough power and influence to be able to help you; be sure that they can devote the time to you; do not choose somebody that has just begun a new job, they will probably not have the time to help you; choose a person with good communication skills who is respected in the organization. It is probably better to choose someone who is not in your direct line of management.

Mentorship is in itself a complete subject, and the benefits for the mentor and mentored are enormous. The mentor gains a supporter and some assistance, the mentored person gains the help and advice of an experienced individual and maybe the chance to try new things. If you decide to choose someone to help with your career development read *Everybody Needs a Mentor* (Clutterbuck 1987). The subject is far too vast to discuss in detail within this volume, but one worth bringing to the attention of anyone who is interested in their own career.

REFERENCE

Clutterbuck D (1987) *Everybody Needs a Mentor.* London: Institute of Personnel Management.

USEFUL READING

Peters T & Waterman R (1982) *In Search of Excellence.* New York: Harper and Row.

8

Funding and Finance

Perhaps the most desirable way of funding activities is to have the financial support of your present employer. In reality, funding from employers is becoming harder to attract as more people are requesting development opportunities and organizations are feeling the squeeze of cost-cutting exercises. The alternatives are to pay for it yourself, raise the money through loans/sales of possessions or to apply to some of the many charitable and business organizations that give grants and awards every year.

The Educational Grants Directory (Eastwood & Casson 1992), available in most libraries, contains details of hundreds of organizations that can be approached directly for support. The *Directory* lists the sources in National and Regional sections; all these bodies award grants for further and higher education and professional development programmes. Details of the contact person, address and conditions of application are outlined. Each year in excess of seventeen million pounds are granted by national sources and a further five million pounds by local sources. Mature students, visits, exchanges and vocational studies are just some of the activities supported.

Currently, the government's Career Development Loan Scheme offers some help for students. One of three banks (Barclays, Cooperative and Clydesdale Bank) can offer you loans of up to eighty per cent of the course costs. The minimum loan is three hundred pounds and the maximum loan is five thousand pounds. Repayments of the loan need not start until three months after the course completion. No interest is charged to the borrower and the government pay the interest charges as part of the scheme. The course must be no longer than one year in length, undertaken in the United Kingdom and be work related (although the work may not necessarily be your current occupation). Contact the participating banks for full details of this scheme and government support along with details of the bank's requirements from applicants.

Some Health Authorities have special trustees or funds which can be applied for through formal channels. This funding can extend to cover not only education and training, but projects and experiences. Most personnel offices will be able to help you pinpoint local sources of finance, such as special trustees.

Most of the major providers of education and training such as the Open University, further education colleges and professional organizations have advisers who are able to discuss your particular financial situation with you and refer you to sources that they particularly attract funding from for students.

PROJECTS, RESEARCH AND EXPERIENCES

Some funding for projects, research and experiences can be funded by sources mentioned in *The Educational Grants Directory* (Eastwood & Casson 1992). Other funding can be attracted from open competition. The nursing press frequently advertise awards for individuals who are interested in developing practice and research. Such awards are gained by open competition and include the *Nursing Times* 3M Award and others such as the Lord Trafford Renal Nursing Award and the Florence Nightingale Memorial Award. Some competitions lead to exchange visits and other experiences of a practical nature.

The speculative approach can be useful if you have a particularly interesting project that you wish to develop. Charitable organizations that do not currently offer regular grants/funding may respond to a request that concerns their particular interest. If you wish to undertake a project which could help an organization, consider approaching them for support. *The Health Directory* (MacDonald 1990) lists voluntary organizations with special interests. *The Hospitals and Health Services Year Book* (Coad 1992) publishes details of organizations that have affiliations with the health services.

Apply to your current employer for assistance with finance, particularly if the project or experience will help to improve the service currently on offer.

EMPLOYMENT

Self-employed status and setting up in business are situations that need discussion with an accountant. A good accountant will be able to guide you through a business plan and help you to attract the right kind of funding for your course of action. Nearly all other forms of employment are paid, with the exception of voluntary work. In some instances all expenses are paid by the voluntary worker's employer; in other instances, the volunteer has to pay some of the costs. If the particular project/work that attracts you does not cover costs the employer will usually be able to advise you about sources of funding. Before you enter into a contract of employment in which you will be expected to pay some of the costs be sure to have identified all of the funds first.

OTHER SOURCES OF FUNDING

Most local public libraries will have details of particular funds and organizations that exist within your region and should be able to help you with addresses for major sources of funding. The Royal College of Nursing administer a small number of funds, details of which are freely available from the RCN.

The Directory of Social Change publishes a comprehensive number of volumes that list thousands of sources of funding amounting to millions of pounds each year. Details of these volumes can be obtained from the Directory of Social Change or your local public library.

APPLYING FOR FUNDING

Many of the sources of funding will have a set method of application, details of which will be sent to you upon request along with details about the amount of money that can be applied for and any terms or conditions. Some charities, individuals or companies may invite applications by letter or proposal. If this is the case, set out your application very clearly and carefully. Send a typed copy. Any letter of application or proposal should include details of the following.

- The nature of the project, experience, training/education.
- Who will benefit and how.
- The expected outcome, e.g., change in practice, new evidence, a degree.
- The time span involved.
- Estimated costs.
- The skills that you have to offer and those you will acquire as a result of undertaking the project.
- Any other resources required and how you intend to provide them.

Each application for funding will vary according to the requirements of the funding body and the details of the project that funding is required for. It is therefore useful to consult an academic who is used to applying for funding. Your nurse tutor or manager may be able to suggest somebody. Most Regional Health Authorities have research nurses who may be able to provide you with some assistance or refer you to local help.

Before you apply for and accept any form of funding make sure that the terms and conditions of the funding are compatible with the professional code of conduct and that the venture itself is ethically sound. If you are at all uncertain contact the UKCC advice lines.

REFERENCES

Coad H (ed) (1992) *The Hospitals and Health Services Yearbook*. London: Institute of Health Services Management.
Eastwood M & Casson D (1992) *The Educational Grants Directory*, 2nd edn. London: Directory of Social Change.
MacDonald F (1990) *The Health Directory*. London: Bedford Square Press.

USEFUL READING

Casson D (ed) (1991) *The Major Companies Guide*, 2nd edn. London: Directory of Social Change.
Clamp G (ed) (1991) *Resources for Nursing Research*. London: Library Association Publication.
Clarke S (1992) *The Complete Fundraising Handbook*. London: Directory of Social Change.
Department of Education (1986) *Career Development Loans (PP855)*. London: Department of Education.
Department of Education (1991) *Sponsorships 1991*. London: Department of Education.
Eastwood M & Casson D (1992) *The Educational Grants Directory*. London: Directory of Social Change.
EGAS (1991) *Money to Study*. London: National Union of Students and Overseas Development Administration.
Family Welfare Association (1991) *Charities Digest*. London: Families Welfare Association.
Fitzherbert L & Forrester S (1991) *A Guide to the Major Trusts*, 3rd edn. London: Directory of Social Change.
Norton M (1989a) *Raising Money from Trusts*. London: Directory of Social Change.
Norton M (1989b) *How to Write Better Fundraising Applications*. London: Directory of Social Change.

Institute of Nursing (1991) *Directory of Funding for Nurses.* Oxford: Institute of Nursing.

USEFUL ADDRESSES

Barclays Bank,
  45 Lombard Street, London EC3P 3AH.
Clydesdale Bank,
  448 Union Street, Aberdeen AB1 1TS.
Cooperative Bank,
  Head Office, PO Box 101, 1 Ballon Street, Manchester M60 4EP.
Department of Education and Science,
  Publications Despatch Centre, Honeypot Lane, Canons Park, Stanmore, Middlesex HA7 1AZ.
Department of Education,
  Dept CW, ISCWO5, The Paddock, Frizinghall, Bradford BD9 4HD.
Department of Education Northern Ireland,
  Rathgael House, Balloo Road, Bangor, Co Down, Northern Ireland BT19 7PR.
Directory of Social Change,
  Radius Works, Back Lane, London NW3 1HL.
EGAS
  c/o Family Welfare Association, 501–505 Kingsland Road, Dalston, London E8 4AU.
Open University,
  Walton Hall, Milton Keynes, MK7 6AB.
Royal College of Nursing,
  20 Cavendish Square, London W1M 0AB.
Scottish Office Education Department,
  Gyleview House, 3 Redheughs Rigg, South Gyle, Edinburgh EH12 9HH.

SPECIFIC CHARITIES AND FUNDING BODIES

Charities and funds that are available to nurses vary according to local and national availability each year. New funds are being added to the list and funds that have finished are being removed on a regular basis. In addition to the large number of funds that are available to nurses anywhere in the British Isles there are smaller, specific local charities and funds. Further details of these can be obtained from local libraries and colleges of nursing.

Nationally available funds have specific criteria for applicants, which need to be ascertained before an application is made.

TRAVEL

Further details about funds for travel can be obtained from the organizations listed below. In many instances the awards are given to work- or experience-related projects which will benefit the workplace or the discipline as well as the individual.

Arthritis and Rheumatism Council Education Trust,
  Arthritis and Rheumatism Council, 41 Eagle Street, London WC1R 4AR.
London and Provincial Nursing Services Award,
  London and Provincial Nursing Services, Head Office, 76 Borough High Street, London SE1 1LL.
National Association of Theatre Nurses Award for Members,
  National Association of Theatre Nurses, 22 Mount Parade, Harrogate, Yorkshire HG1 1BV.
National Florence Nightingale Memorial Awards,
  National Florence Nightingale Memorial Committee, 6 Grosvenor Crescent, London SW1.
Nuffield Foundation Fellowships,
  The Director, 28 Bedford Square, London WC1B 3EG.
Nurofen Pain Relief Project,
  4–5 Cloisters House, 8 Battersea Park Road, London SW8 4BG.
Psoriasis Association/Josie Bradbury Travel Award,
  The Psoriasis Association, 7 Milton Street, Northampton NN2 7JG.
Royal National Pension Fund/RCN Travel Scholarship,
  Royal College of Nursing, 20 Cavendish Square, London W1M 0AB.
The Commonwealth Foundation,
  The Director, Marlborough House, Pall Mall, London SW19 5HY.
The Commonwealth Youth Exchange Council,
  The Executive Secretary, 18 Fleet Street, London EC4Y 1AA.
The Florence and Don McGregor Trust,
  c/o Maurice Plaskow, 9 Lakeside, Oatlands Drive, Weybridge, Surrey KT13 9JB.
The Harkness Fellowship,
  28 Bedford Square, London WC1B 3EG.
The Winston Churchill Memorial Trust Fund,
  c/o Sir Richard Vickers, Director General, 15 Queen's Gate Terrace, London SW7 5PR.

PRACTICE DEVELOPMENT AND RESEARCH

Each of the individual organizations listed below have different criteria for applicants. Often the criteria are related to the organization's special interest.

Action for Dysphasic Adults,
    Northcote House, 37a Royal Street, London SE1 7LL.
Alcohol Education and Research Council,
    Abell House (RMG6), John Islip Street, London SW1P 4LH.
Association for Spina Bifida and Hydrocephalus,
    22 Upper Woburn Place, London WC1H 0HP.
Birthright/Evian Bursaries,
    Birthright, 27 Sussex Place, Regents Park, London NW1 4SP.
Birthright/Royal College of Gynaecologists,
    27 Sussex Place, Regents Park, London NW1 4SP.
British Commonwealth Nurses War Memorial Fund,
    20 Brunswick Road, London E10 6RS.
British Migraine Association,
    178a High Road, Byfleet, Weybridge, Surrey KT14 7ED.
Cancer Relief/MacMillan Fund,
    Anchor House, 15–19 Britten Street, London SW3 3TZ.
Cancer Research Campaign,
    2 Carlton House Terrace, London SW1Y 5AR.
Child Growth Foundation,
    2 Mayfield Avenue, Chiswick, London W4 1PW.
Community Outlook/3M Pathfinder Award,
    Nursing Times, Macmillan Magazines Ltd, 4 Little Essex Street, London WC2R 3LF.
Elizabeth Clark Charitable Trust for Nurses,
    c/o Miss Vera Darling, 9 Red Lion Court, London EC4A 3EB.
Foundation for the Study of Infant Deaths,
    Scientific Advisory Committee, 15 Belgrave Square, London SW1X 8PS.
Foundation of Nursing Studies,
    154 Buckingham Palace Road, London SW1 9TR.
Health Services Management Development Trust,
    Institute of Health Services Management, 75 Portland Place, London W1N 4AN.
Lederele Award for Innovation in Cancer Care,
    Awards Coordinator, Brands House, Kingshill Road, High Wycombe, Bucks.
Leverhulme Trust Scholarships and Grants,
    Research Awards Committee, The Leverhulme Trust, 15–19 Fetter Lane, London EC4A 1NR.

London and Provincial Nursing Services Awards,
    Head Office, 76 Borough High Street, London SE1 1LL.
Maws Midwives Research Scholarships,
    Maws, 50 Upper Brook Street, London W1Y 1PG.
Muscular Dystrophy Group (Grants),
    Natrass House, 35 Macaulay Road, London SW4 0QP.
National Association of Theatre Nurses,
    22 Mount Parade, Harrogate, Yorkshire HG1 1BV.
National Back Pain Association,
    31–33 Park Road, Teddington, Middlesex TW11 0AB.
Novo Nordisk,
    Broadfield Park, Brighton Road, Pease Cottage, Crawley, West Sussex
    RH11 9RT.
Nursing Standard/Awards,
    Nursing Standard, 17–19 Peterborough Road, Harrow HA1 2AX.
Queens Nursing Institute Awards,
    The Queens Nursing Institute, 3 Albermarle Way, London EC1V
    4JB.
Royal College of Midwives Trust,
    15 Mansfield Street, London W1M 0BE.
Royal College of Nursing,
    20 Cavendish Square, London W1M 0AB.
The Trevor Clay Trust,
    c/o The Royal College of Nursing (see above).
Wyeth Laboratories Female Health Care Award,
    Wyeth Laboratories, Huntercombe Lane South, Taplow, Maidenhead,
    Berks SL6 0PH.

EDUCATION AND TRAINING

The organizations listed in this section give awards that range from
small amounts for individual study sessions to grants for full courses.
Some organizations only sponsor education and training that is relevant to their own special interest. Others have few specific restrictions
and criteria. As is the case with all the organizations listed in this
section on funding, the criteria may be subject to change from time
to time.

Alcohol Education and Research Council,
    Abell House (RM G6), John Islip Street, London SW1P 4LH.
Arthritis and Rheumatism Council,
    Junior and Senior Postgraduate Awards, 41 Eagle Street, London
    WC1R 4AR.
Ashbourne Hill Management College Bursary,

Ashbourne Hill College, Ashbourne Hill, Leamington Spa, Warwickshire CV33 9QW.

Band Trust Scholarships (Research Methodology),
c/o The Florence Nightingale Memorial Trust, The National Florence Nightingale Memorial Committee, 9 Grosvenor Crescent, London SW1X 7EH.

British Association of Health Services in Higher Education,
University Health Centre, Northcourt Avenue, Reading, Berks RG2 7HE.

British Commonwealth Nurses War Memorial Fund,
20 Brunswick Road, London E10 6RS.

British Geriatric Society (Study Grants),
1 St Andrews Place, Regents Park, London NW1 4LB.

Career Development Loans,
c/o Barclays Bank, Cooperative Bank, Clydesdale Bank, Department of Employment. Details are available from any of these organizations.

Economic and Social Research Council,
Cherry Orchard East, Kembrey Park, Swindon, Wiltshire SN2 6UQ.

Health Services Management Development Trust,
Institute of Health Services Management, 75 Portland Place, London W1N 4AN.

Noah Trust,
15 Blenheim Road, London NW8 0LU.

Royal College of Nursing,
20 Cavendish Square, London W1M 0AB.

Scottish Home Office and Health Department,
Chief Scientist Office, Room 207, St Andrews House, Edinburgh EH1 3DE.

Sidney Perry Foundation,
Atlas Assurance Company, Trustee Department, Civic Drive, Ipswich IP1 2AN.

Sir Richard Stapley Educational Trust,
1 York Street, London W1H 1PZ.

Students Loans Company Ltd,
100 Bothwell Street, Glasgow G2 7JD.

St John Ambulance Nursing Bursaries,
St John Headquarters, 1 Grosvenor Crescent, London SW1X 7EF.

The Department of Health Research Training Awards,
Quarry House, Quarry Hill, Leeds, Yorkshire LS2 7UD.

The Elizabeth Nuffield Educational Fund,
The Secretary to the Committee, 28 Bedford Square, London WC1B 3EG.

The Gilchrist Educational Trust,
  The Secretary, International Students House, 229 Great Portland Street, London W1N 5HD.
The Grantham Yorke Trust,
  c/o The Clerk, 41 Church Street, Birmingham B3 2DY.
The Laura Ashley Foundation,
  Dr John Rae, 31 Old Burlington Street, London W1X 1LB.
The London and Provincial Nursing Service Awards,
  Head Office, 76 Borough High Street, London SE1 1LL.
The Lord Ashdown Charitable Settlement,
  c/o Clive Marks and Company, 44a New Cavendish Street, London W1M 7LG.
The Mary MacArthur Educational Trust,
  c/o The Secretary, Central House, Upper Woburn Place, London WC1H 0HY.
The Nancy Balfour Trust,
  c/o Messrs Sayers Butterworth, 18 Bentinck Street, London W1M 5RL.
The Smith and Nephew Foundation,
  Barbara Bash, Smith and Nephew, Gilston Park, Harlow, Essex CM20 2RQ.
The Society of Apothecaries General Charity,
  The Clerk, Apothecaries Hall, Blackfriars Lane, London EC4V 6EJ.
The Society for Promoting the Training of Women,
  The Secretary, The Deans Cottages, Village Lane, Hedgerley, Slough SL2 3UY.
Women's Careers Foundation,
  The Secretary, 2 Watch Oak, Blackham, Tunbridge Wells, Kent TN3 9TP.

Appendix 1

Name

Permanent address

Telephone no.   **Home:**   **Work**

Education

(List your schools, colleges and higher education. Give dates of attendance. Usually your last experience is the first to be listed.)

Qualifications gained

(List your qualifications detailing the grades and dates that they were obtained.)

Previous employment

(In date order list your previous employment. Make sure that there are no periods in time that are unaccounted for. List employment in the same date order that your education and qualifications are listed. Reflect upon your experiences and list any special skills and knowledge that you have gained or contributed to each experience.)

Current employment

(Detail your current employment including particular responsibilities and contributions to the job. Reflect upon skills and knowledge gained while in post, especially those items that are relevant to the post applied for.)

Referees

(Give the names and addresses of three referees. Gain the consent of the referees first.)

Appendix 2

An example of a pre-interview checklist given as guidance to second level nurses being interviewed for the conversion course.

CHECKLIST (1) YOU AS INTERVIEWEE

Areas you may wish to consider prior to coming to interview.

A Your expertise

(i) *Clinical*

- Special skills.
- Areas in which you have a particular interest.
- Any studies/research that you have done.

(ii) *Management*

- Any occasions when you may have taken charge.
- Any change that you have either instigated or been part of (e.g., introduction of primary nursing).
- The way in which you manage your own daily workload/patient care/time and the work of any other people in your team.

(iii) *Educational*

153

- Responsibility for training others in any capacity – either formal teaching or one-to-one discussion on the job.
- Any particular research that you have done and applied to the practical areas.

B Your education

- Any courses that you have attended.
- Journals that you read to keep up to date.
- Your studies at the moment.

C Why you want to do the course

- Consider your strengths in the clinical, education and managerial fields; use these at this point.
- Understand what the difference is between first and second level nurses so that you can explain what it is that the course will give you that you do not already have – what it will further develop.
- Consider your future plans as an individual and as a nurse.
- Let them know what you have to offer.

D Why you should have a place as opposed to all the other excellent candidates

- Your commitment to further development. Study that you have undertaken in your own time and other examples.
- Consider everything that you have done to date that has helped to improve patient care.
- Your commitment to the profession – lack of sickness absence, attendance record, etc.
- Spell out areas that you have already started to work on that are part of a first level nurse's role, with regard to management of change, management of others. Development of clinical care.
- Your future career plans and progression.

E Understand the difference between the traditional first level training and the P2000 training

- Consider how you might fit in with the P2000 student.
- Understand P2000.

F Read and understand PREP

G Consider current Health Service issues

CHECKLIST (2) UNDERSTAND THE INTERVIEW PANEL

Before you come to interview remember that the panel are not trying to catch you out; they are simply trying to make a difficult choice.

They will naturally have a number of things that will be important to them which you may wish to consider when thinking about their questions.

- Will you be able to cope with the academic work?
- Will you benefit from the course?
- What will you give back to the service if they send you on the course?
- Are you first level material?
- Do you know what the new role would encompass?
- Are you going to complete the course?
- What are your future plans?
- What is your track record to date?

They may not ask these questions, and others, directly but the thoughts will be in their minds, so try to put these at rest by using the things you have considered about yourself.

Appendix 3

Department of Health,
  Quarry House, Quarry Hill, Leeds, Yorkshire LS2 7UD.
Department of Health, Northern Ireland,
  Dundonald House, Upper Newtownards Road, Belfast BT4 3SB.
English National Board Resource and Careers Service,
  PO Box 356, Sheffield S8 0SJ.
King's Fund Centre,
  126 Albert Street, London NW1 7NF.
Nurses Central Clearing House,
  PO Box 346, Bristol BS99 7FB.
Royal College of Nursing of the United Kingdom,
  20 Cavendish Square, London W1M 0AB.
Royal College of Nursing,
  17 Windsor Avenue, Belfast, Northern Ireland.
Royal College of Nursing,
  Tŷ Maeth, King George V Drive East, Cardiff CF4 4XZ.
Royal College of Nursing,
  Glenbourne House, 42 South Oswald Road, Edinburgh EH9 2HH.
Scottish Home and Health Department,
  St Andrews House, Regent Road, Edinburgh EH1 3DE.
The English National Board for Nursing Midwifery and Health
  Visiting,
  Victory House, 170 Tottenham Court Road, London W1P 0HA.
The National Board for Nursing Midwifery and Health Visiting in
  Scotland,
  22 Queen Street, Edinburgh EH2 1JX.

The National Board for Nursing Midwifery and Health Visiting, Northern Ireland,
RAC House, 79 Chichester Street, Belfast BT1 4JR.
The Welsh National Board for Nursing Midwifery and Health Visiting,
13th Floor, Pearl Assurance House, Greyfriars Street, Cardiff CF1 3AG.
United Kingdom Central Council for Nursing Midwifery and Health Visiting,
23 Portland Place, London W1N 3AF.

Index